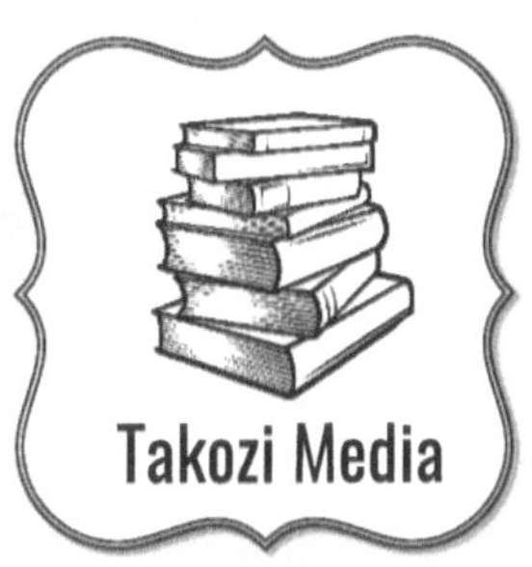

Takozi Media

I0791168

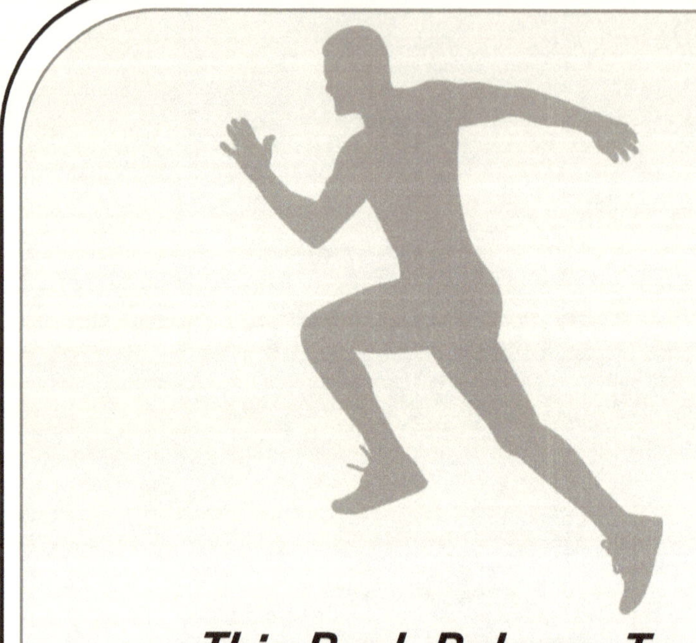

This Book Belongs To:

....

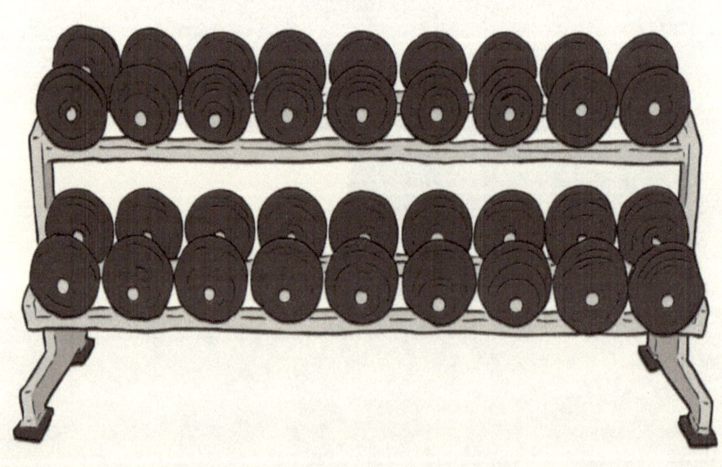

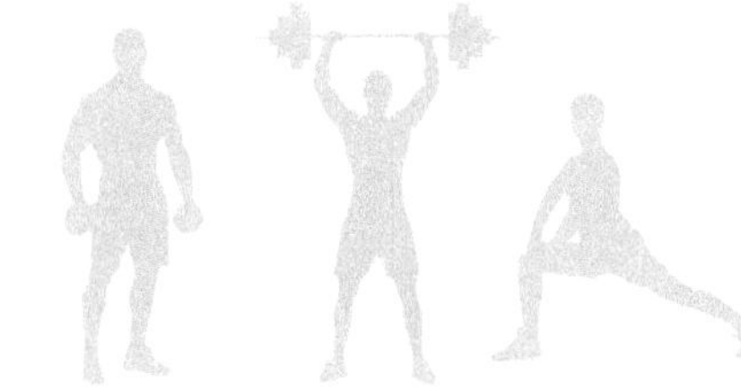

Name: ....

Date: ....

Time: ....

Warm-Up

ACTIVITY	TIME	REPS

Cardio

ACTIVITY	DISTANCE	TIME	TARGET HEART RATE

Strength Training

EXERCISE	SET ONE WEIGHT/REPS	SET TWO WEIGHT/REPS	SET THREE WEIGHT/REPS

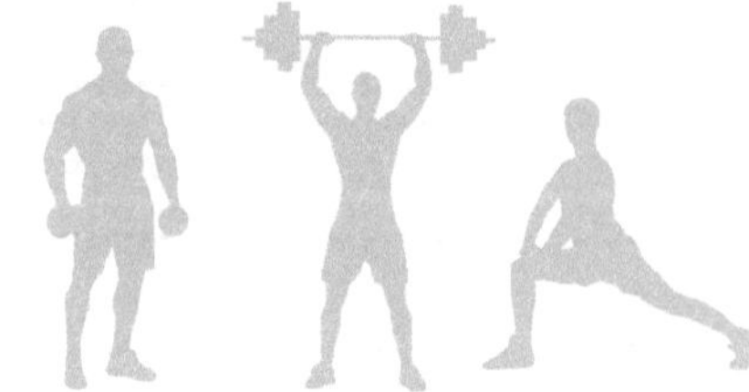

Name: ....

Date: ....

Time: ....

Warm-Up

ACTIVITY	TIME	REPS

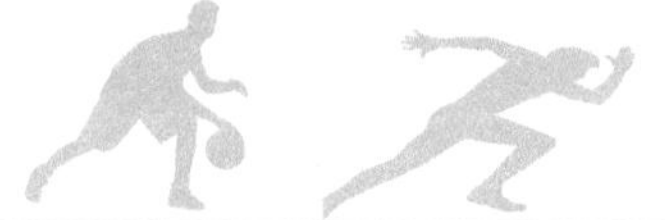 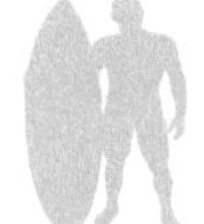 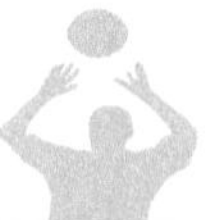 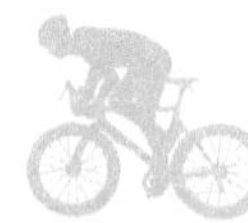

Cardio

ACTIVITY	DISTANCE	TIME	TARGET HEART RATE

Strength Training

EXERCISE	SET ONE WEIGHT/REPS	SET TWO WEIGHT/REPS	SET THREE WEIGHT/REPS

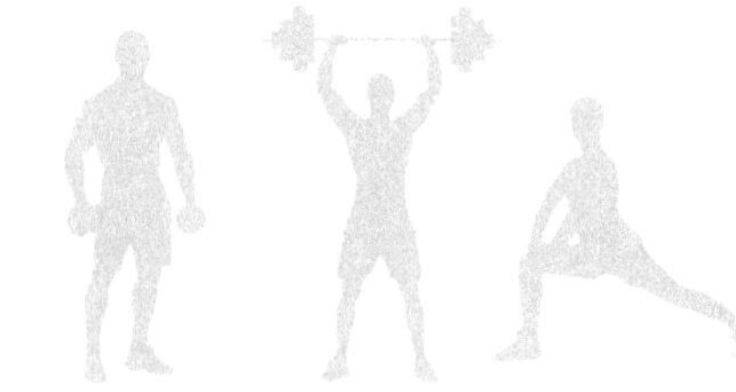

Name: ....

Date: ....

Time: ....

Warm-Up

ACTIVITY	TIME	REPS

Cardio

ACTIVITY	DISTANCE	TIME	TARGET HEART RATE

Strength Training

EXERCISE	SET ONE WEIGHT/REPS	SET TWO WEIGHT/REPS	SET THREE WEIGHT/REPS

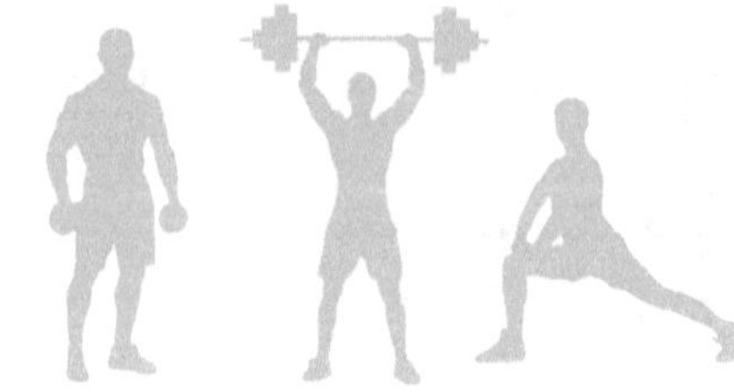

Name: ....

Date: ....

Time: ....

Warm-Up

ACTIVITY	TIME	REPS

 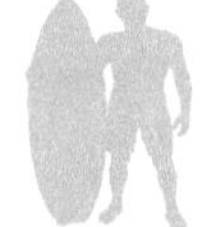 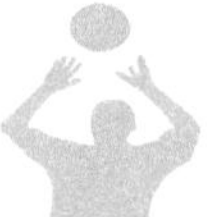 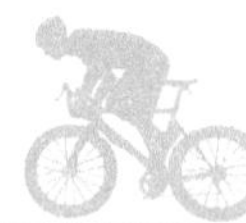

Cardio

ACTIVITY	DISTANCE	TIME	TARGET HEART RATE

Strength Training

EXERCISE	SET ONE WEIGHT/REPS	SET TWO WEIGHT/REPS	SET THREE WEIGHT/REPS

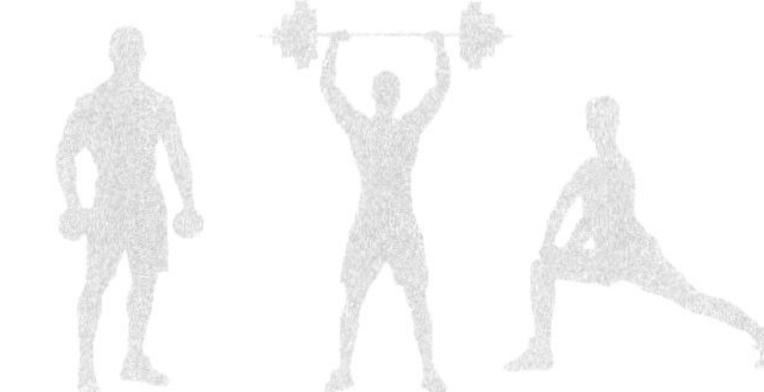

Name: ....

Date: ....

Time: ....

Warm-Up

ACTIVITY	TIME	REPS

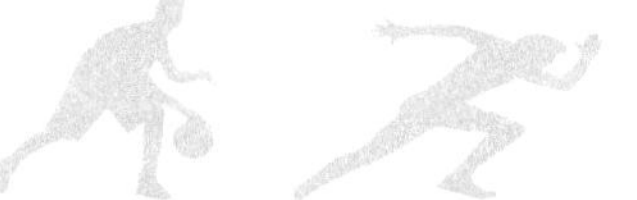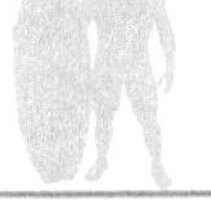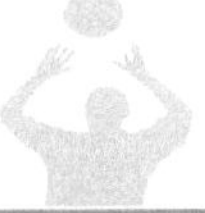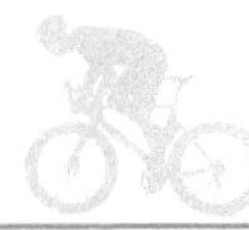

Cardio

ACTIVITY	DISTANCE	TIME	TARGET HEART RATE

Strength Training

EXERCISE	SET ONE WEIGHT/REPS	SET TWO WEIGHT/REPS	SET THREE WEIGHT/REPS

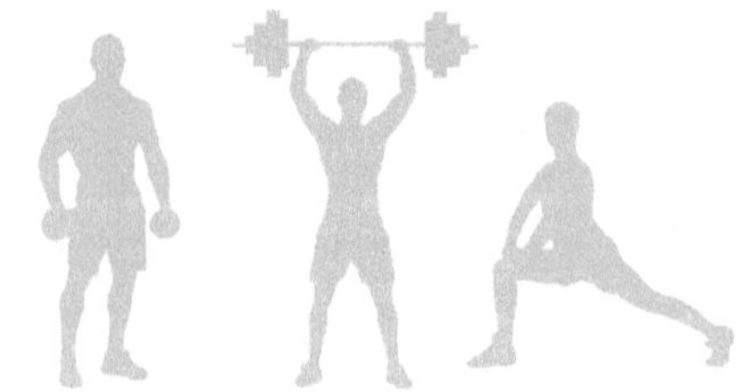

Warm-Up

ACTIVITY	TIME	REPS

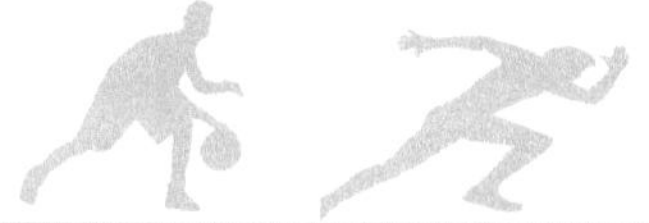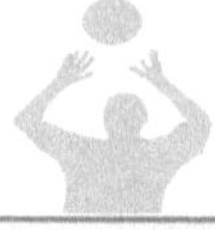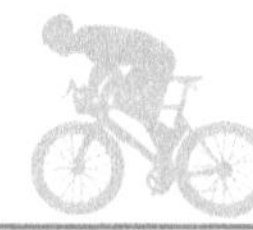

Cardio

ACTIVITY	DISTANCE	TIME	TARGET HEART RATE

Strength Training

EXERCISE	SET ONE WEIGHT/REPS	SET TWO WEIGHT/REPS	SET THREE WEIGHT/REPS

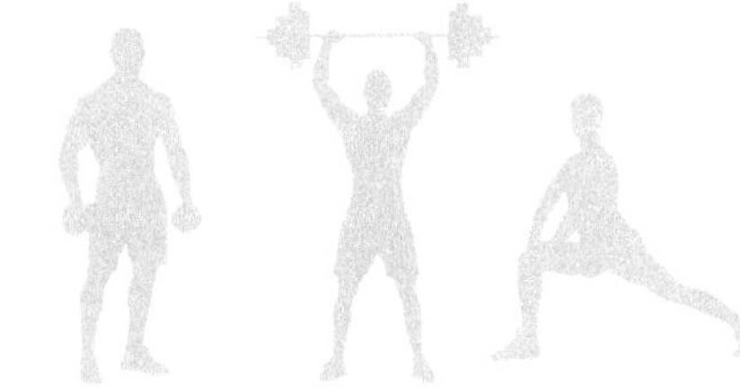

Name: ....

Date: ....

Time: ....

Warm-Up

ACTIVITY	TIME	REPS

Cardio

ACTIVITY	DISTANCE	TIME	TARGET HEART RATE

Strength Training

EXERCISE	SET ONE WEIGHT/REPS	SET TWO WEIGHT/REPS	SET THREE WEIGHT/REPS

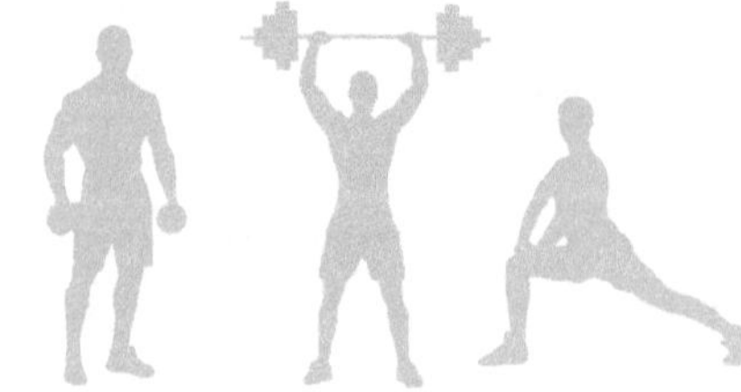

Name: ....

Date: ....

Time: ....

Warm-Up

ACTIVITY	TIME	REPS

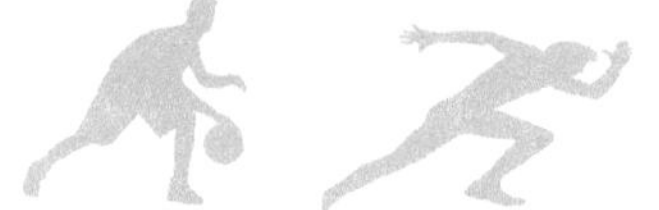 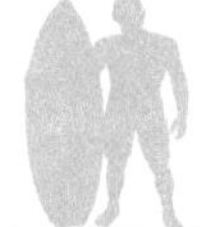 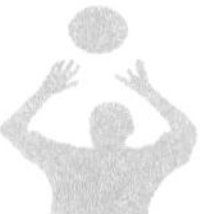 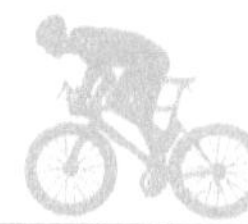

Cardio

ACTIVITY	DISTANCE	TIME	TARGET HEART RATE

Strength Training

EXERCISE	SET ONE WEIGHT/REPS	SET TWO WEIGHT/REPS	SET THREE WEIGHT/REPS

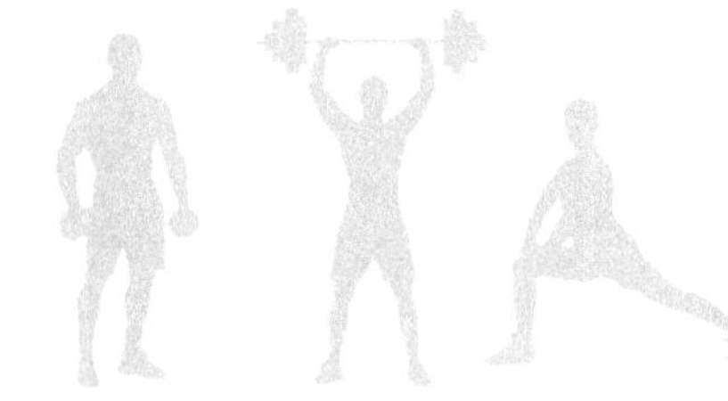

Name: ....

Date: ....

Time: ....

Warm-Up

ACTIVITY	TIME	REPS

Cardio

ACTIVITY	DISTANCE	TIME	TARGET HEART RATE

Strength Training

EXERCISE	SET ONE WEIGHT/REPS	SET TWO WEIGHT/REPS	SET THREE WEIGHT/REPS

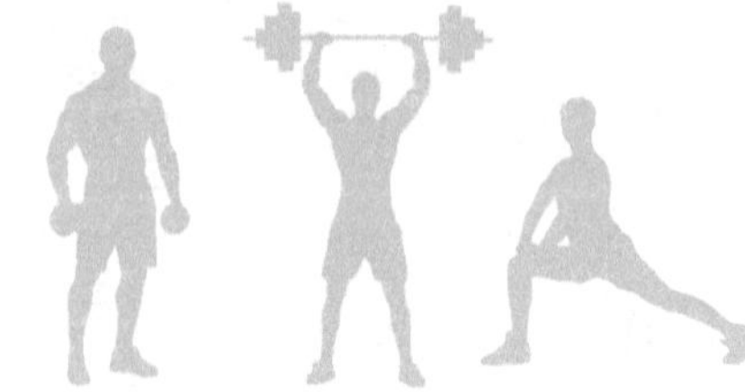

Name: ....

Date: ....

Time: ....

Warm-Up

ACTIVITY	TIME	REPS

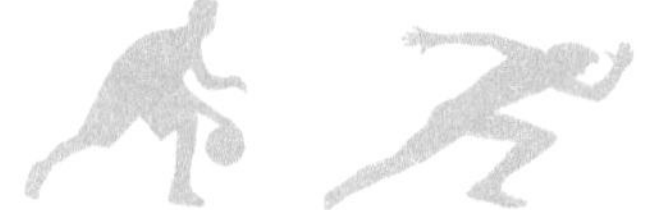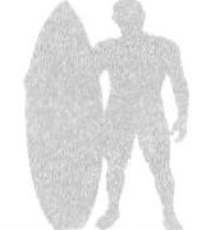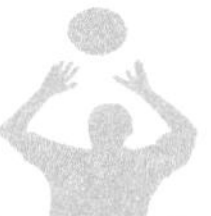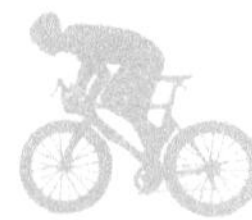

Cardio

ACTIVITY	DISTANCE	TIME	TARGET HEART RATE

Strength Training

EXERCISE	SET ONE WEIGHT/REPS	SET TWO WEIGHT/REPS	SET THREE WEIGHT/REPS

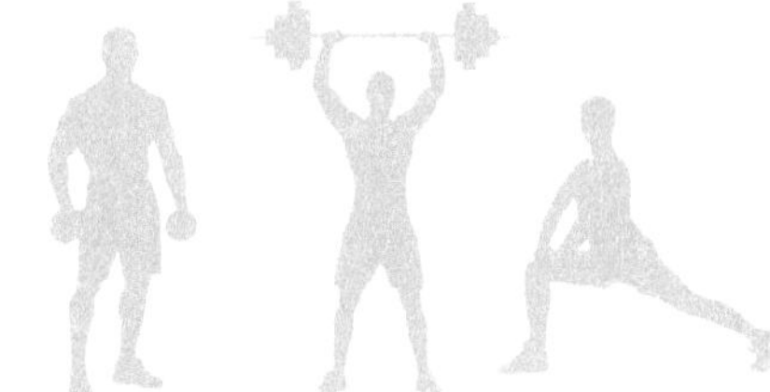

Name: ....

Date: ....

Time: ....

Warm-Up

ACTIVITY	TIME	REPS

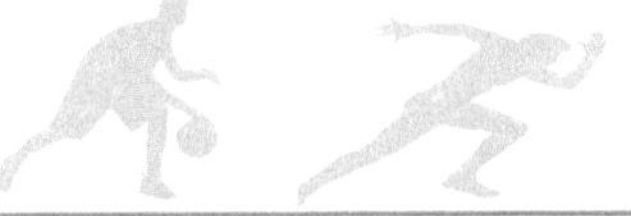 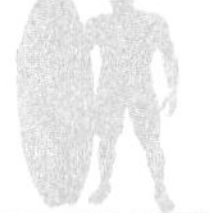 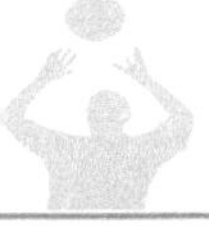 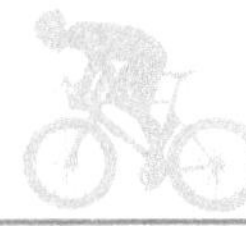

Cardio

ACTIVITY	DISTANCE	TIME	TARGET HEART RATE

Strength Training

EXERCISE	SET ONE WEIGHT/REPS	SET TWO WEIGHT/REPS	SET THREE WEIGHT/REPS

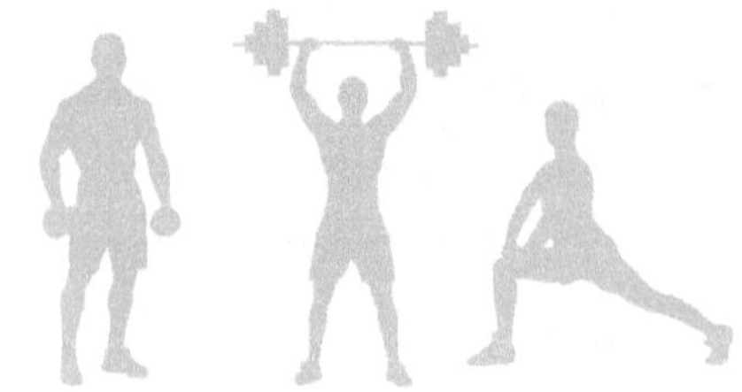

Name: ....

Date: ....

Time: ....

Warm-Up

ACTIVITY	TIME	REPS

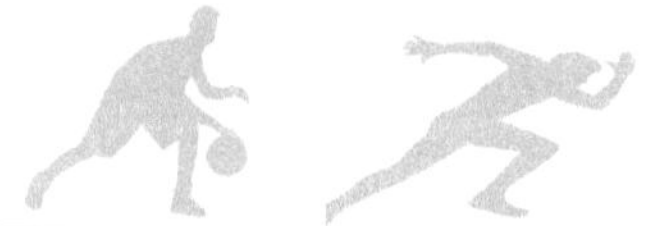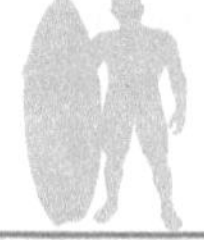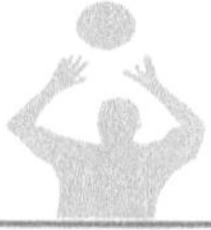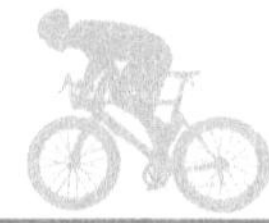

Cardio

ACTIVITY	DISTANCE	TIME	TARGET HEART RATE

Strength Training

EXERCISE	SET ONE WEIGHT/REPS	SET TWO WEIGHT/REPS	SET THREE WEIGHT/REPS

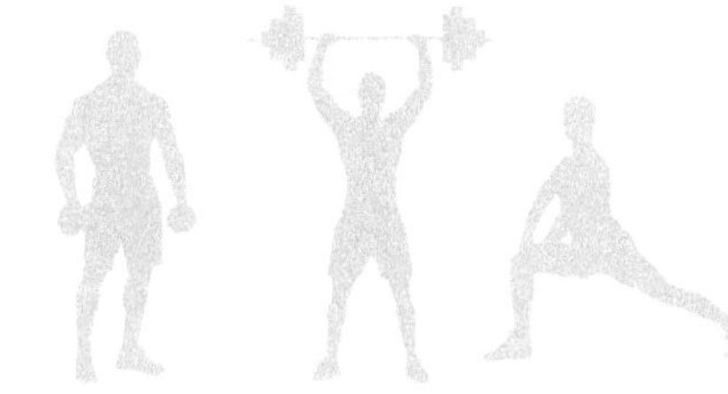

Warm-Up

ACTIVITY	TIME	REPS

Cardio

ACTIVITY	DISTANCE	TIME	TARGET HEART RATE

Strength Training

EXERCISE	SET ONE WEIGHT/REPS	SET TWO WEIGHT/REPS	SET THREE WEIGHT/REPS

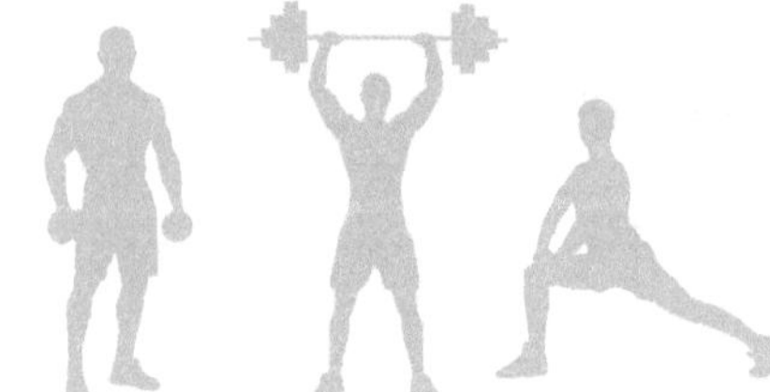

Name: ....

Date: ....

Time: ....

Warm-Up

ACTIVITY	TIME	REPS

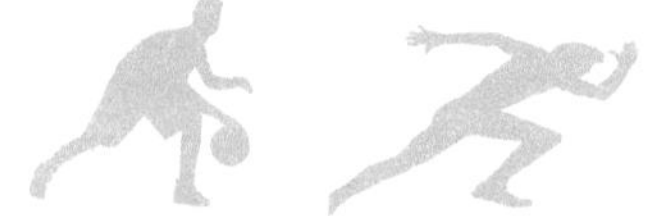 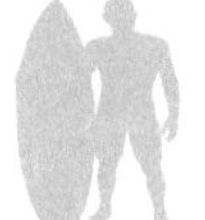 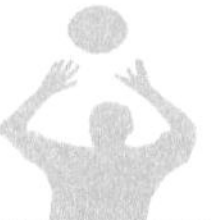 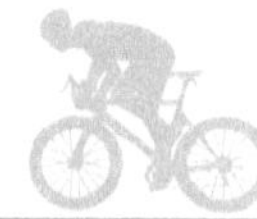

Cardio

ACTIVITY	DISTANCE	TIME	TARGET HEART RATE

Strength Training

EXERCISE	SET ONE WEIGHT/REPS	SET TWO WEIGHT/REPS	SET THREE WEIGHT/REPS

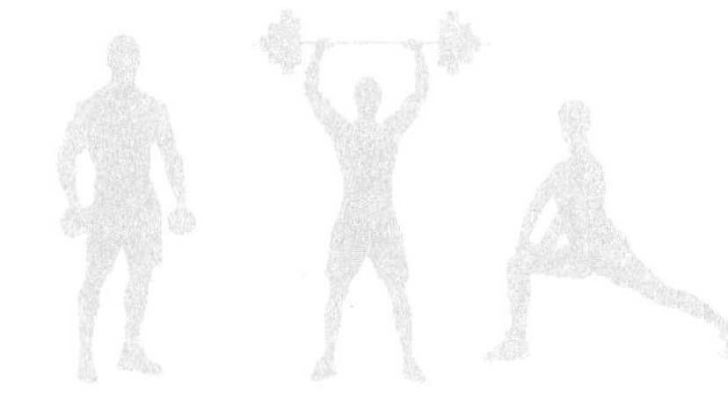

Name: ....

Date: ....

Time: ....

Warm-Up

ACTIVITY	TIME	REPS

Cardio

ACTIVITY	DISTANCE	TIME	TARGET HEART RATE

Strength Training

EXERCISE	SET ONE WEIGHT/REPS	SET TWO WEIGHT/REPS	SET THREE WEIGHT/REPS

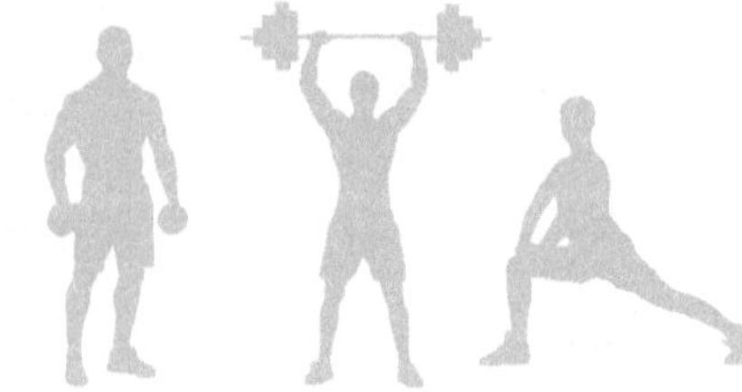

Name: ....

Date: ....

Time: ....

Warm-Up

ACTIVITY	TIME	REPS

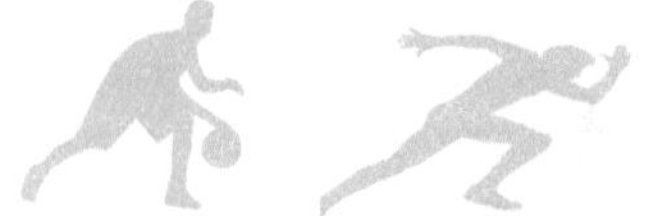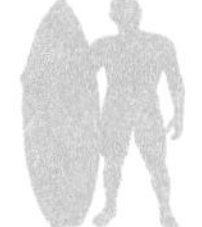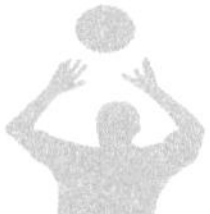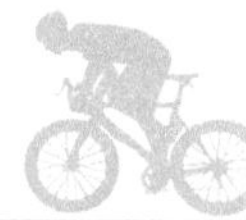

Cardio

ACTIVITY	DISTANCE	TIME	TARGET HEART RATE

Strength Training

EXERCISE	SET ONE WEIGHT/REPS	SET TWO WEIGHT/REPS	SET THREE WEIGHT/REPS

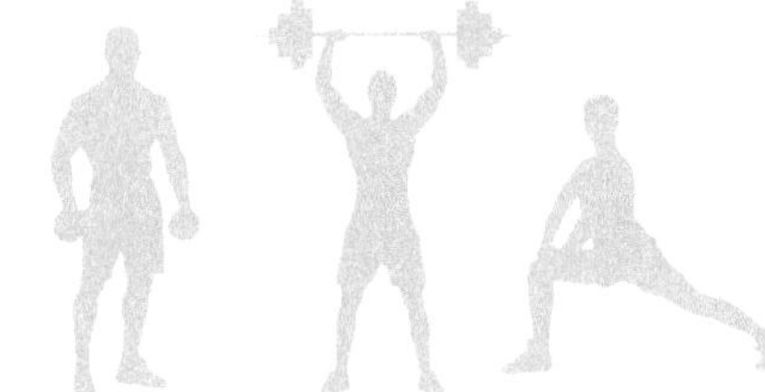

Name: ....

Date: ....

Time: ....

Warm-Up

ACTIVITY	TIME	REPS

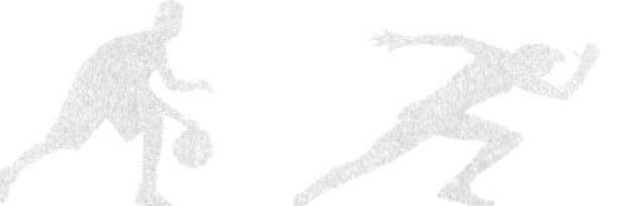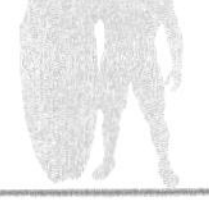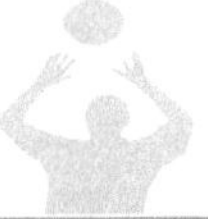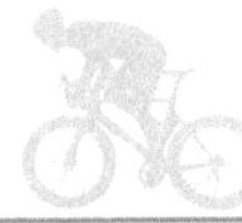

Cardio

ACTIVITY	DISTANCE	TIME	TARGET HEART RATE

Strength Training

EXERCISE	SET ONE WEIGHT/REPS	SET TWO WEIGHT/REPS	SET THREE WEIGHT/REPS

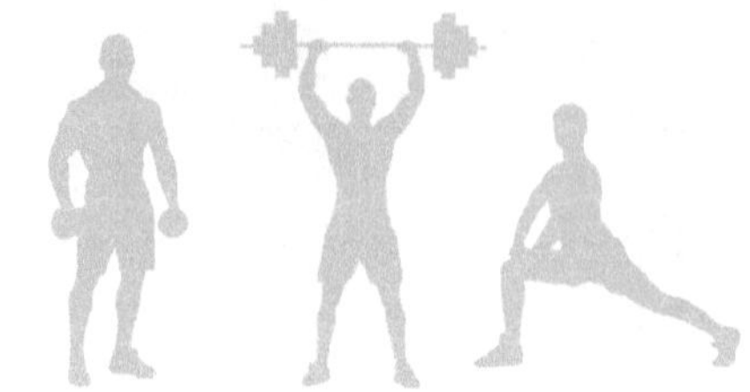

Name: ....

Date: ....

Time: ....

Warm-Up

ACTIVITY	TIME	REPS

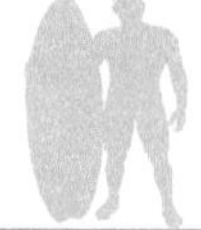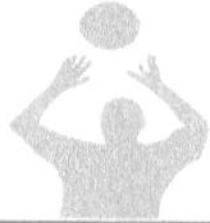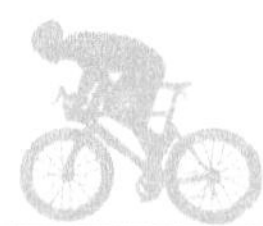

Cardio

ACTIVITY	DISTANCE	TIME	TARGET HEART RATE

Strength Training

EXERCISE	SET ONE WEIGHT/REPS	SET TWO WEIGHT/REPS	SET THREE WEIGHT/REPS

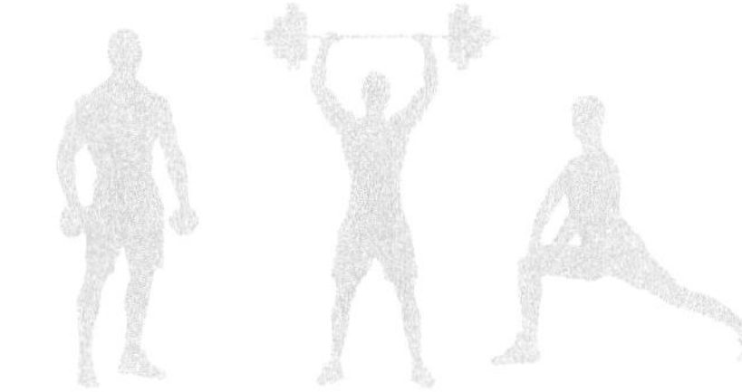

Name: ....

Date: ....

Time: ....

Warm-Up

ACTIVITY	TIME	REPS

Cardio

ACTIVITY	DISTANCE	TIME	TARGET HEART RATE

Strength Training

EXERCISE	SET ONE WEIGHT/REPS	SET TWO WEIGHT/REPS	SET THREE WEIGHT/REPS

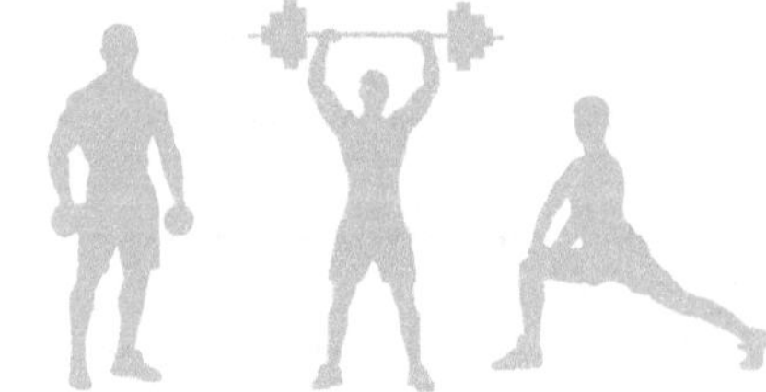

Warm-Up

ACTIVITY	TIME	REPS

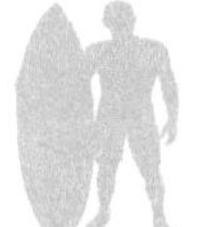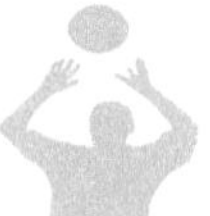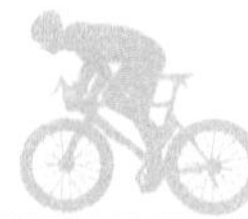

Cardio

ACTIVITY	DISTANCE	TIME	TARGET HEART RATE

Strength Training

EXERCISE	SET ONE WEIGHT/REPS	SET TWO WEIGHT/REPS	SET THREE WEIGHT/REPS

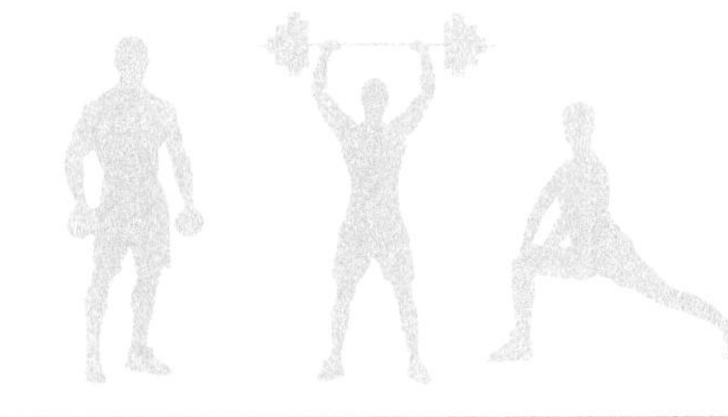

Name: ....

Date: ....

Time: ....

Warm-Up

ACTIVITY	TIME	REPS

Cardio

ACTIVITY	DISTANCE	TIME	TARGET HEART RATE

Strength Training

EXERCISE	SET ONE WEIGHT/REPS	SET TWO WEIGHT/REPS	SET THREE WEIGHT/REPS

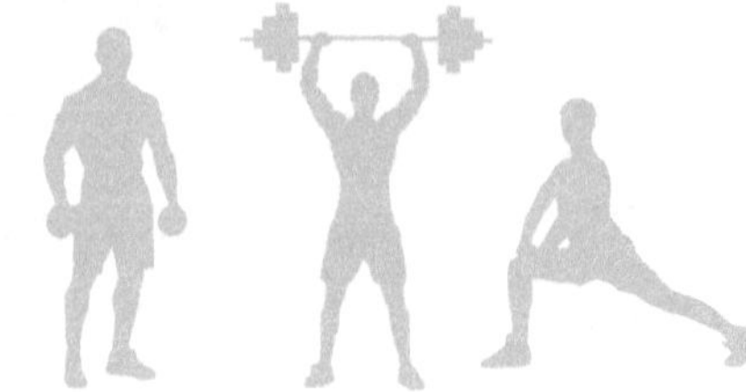

Name: ....

Date: ....

Time: ....

Warm-Up

ACTIVITY	TIME	REPS

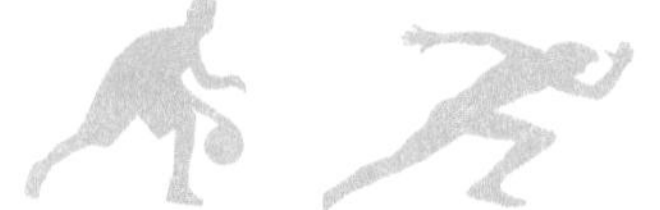 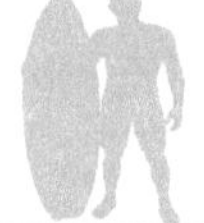 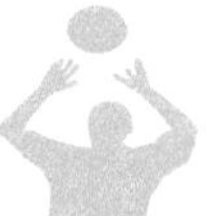 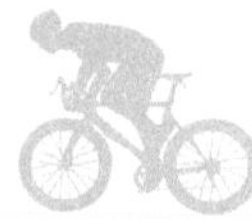

Cardio

ACTIVITY	DISTANCE	TIME	TARGET HEART RATE

Strength Training

EXERCISE	SET ONE WEIGHT/REPS	SET TWO WEIGHT/REPS	SET THREE WEIGHT/REPS

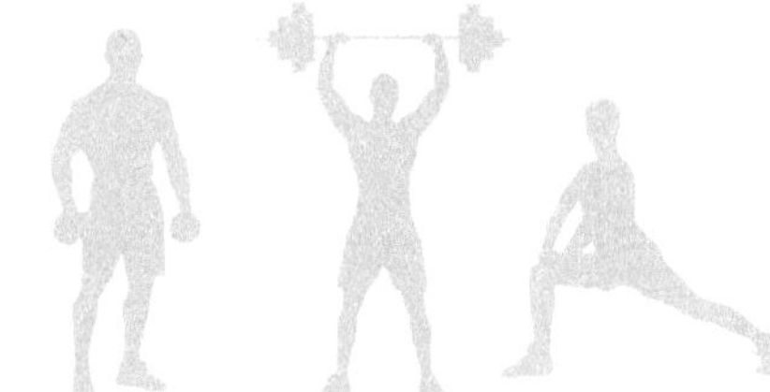

Name: ....

Date: ....

Time: ....

Warm-Up

ACTIVITY	TIME	REPS

 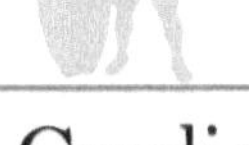 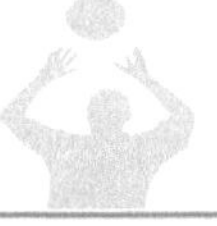 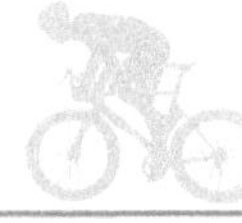

Cardio

ACTIVITY	DISTANCE	TIME	TARGET HEART RATE

Strength Training

EXERCISE	SET ONE WEIGHT/REPS	SET TWO WEIGHT/REPS	SET THREE WEIGHT/REPS

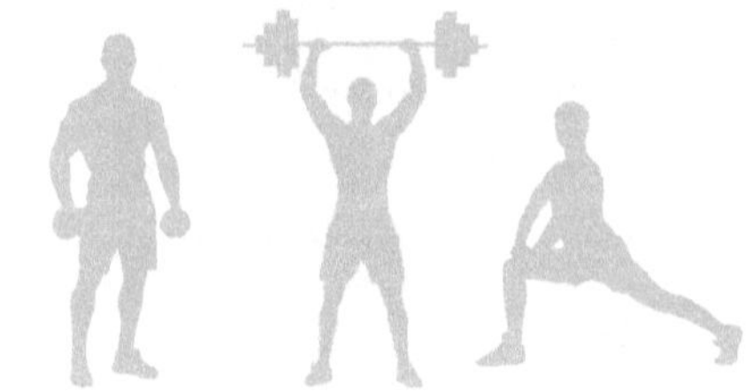

Name: ....

Date: ....

Time: ....

Warm-Up

ACTIVITY	TIME	REPS

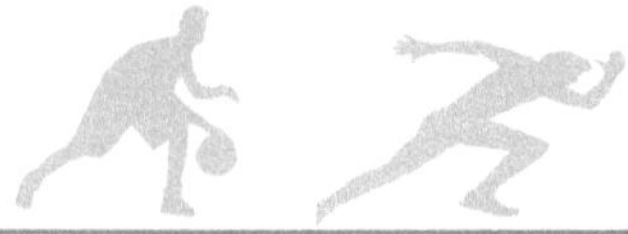 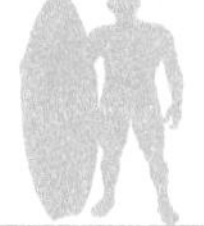 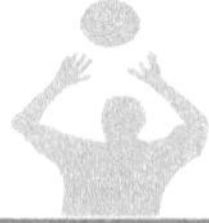 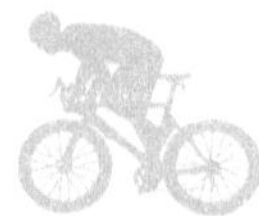

Cardio

ACTIVITY	DISTANCE	TIME	TARGET HEART RATE

Strength Training

EXERCISE	SET ONE WEIGHT/REPS	SET TWO WEIGHT/REPS	SET THREE WEIGHT/REPS

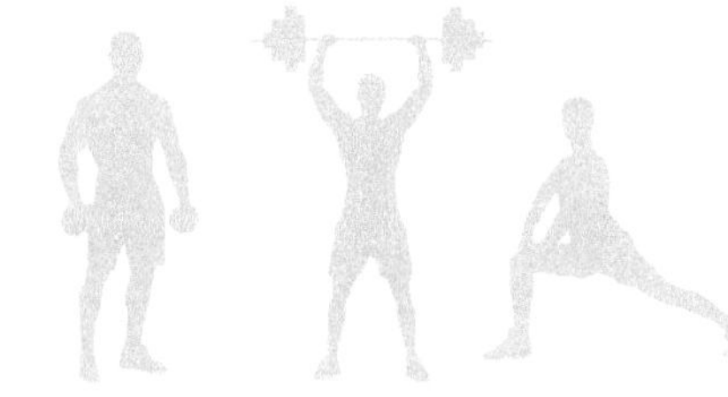

Name: ....

Date: ....

Time: ....

Warm-Up

ACTIVITY	TIME	REPS

Cardio

ACTIVITY	DISTANCE	TIME	TARGET HEART RATE

Strength Training

EXERCISE	SET ONE WEIGHT/REPS	SET TWO WEIGHT/REPS	SET THREE WEIGHT/REPS

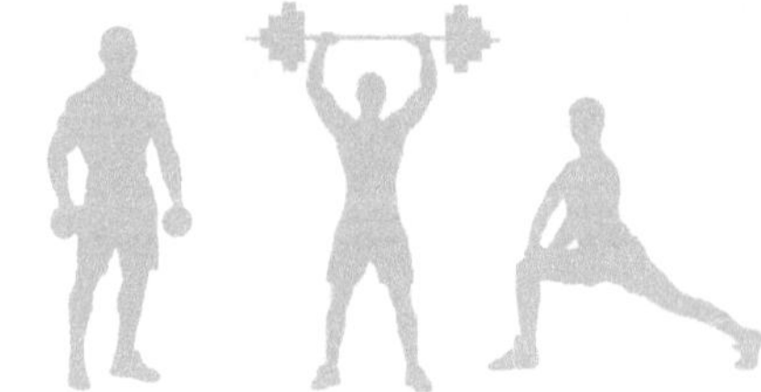

Warm-Up

ACTIVITY	TIME	REPS

 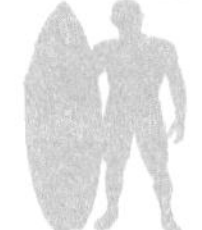 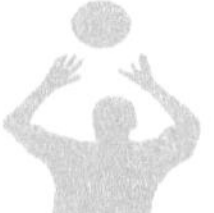 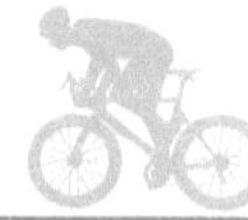

Cardio

ACTIVITY	DISTANCE	TIME	TARGET HEART RATE

Strength Training

EXERCISE	SET ONE WEIGHT/REPS	SET TWO WEIGHT/REPS	SET THREE WEIGHT/REPS

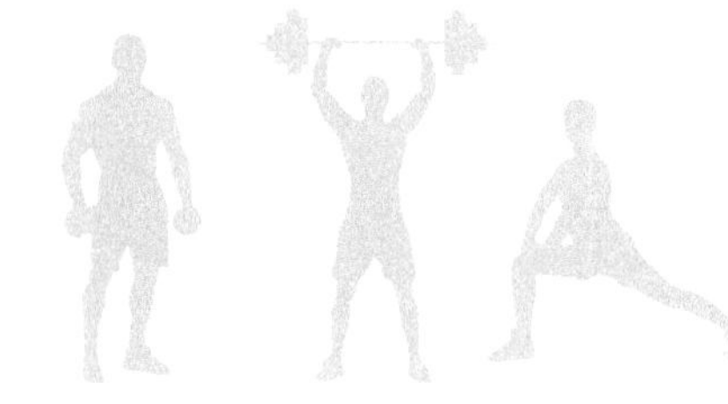

Name: ....

Date: ....

Time: ....

Warm-Up

ACTIVITY	TIME	REPS

Cardio

ACTIVITY	DISTANCE	TIME	TARGET HEART RATE

Strength Training

EXERCISE	SET ONE WEIGHT/REPS	SET TWO WEIGHT/REPS	SET THREE WEIGHT/REPS

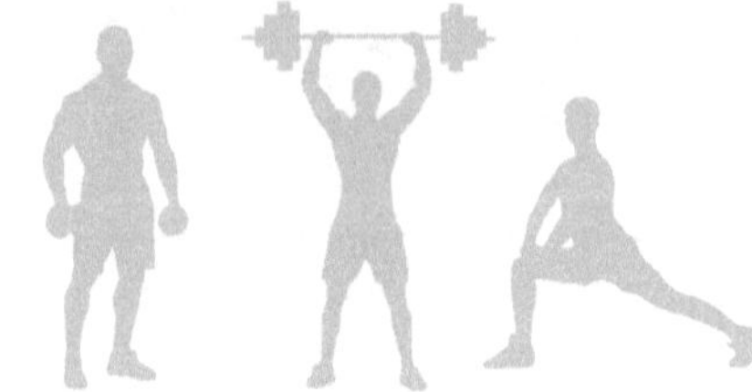

Name: ....

Date: ....

Time: ....

Warm-Up

ACTIVITY	TIME	REPS

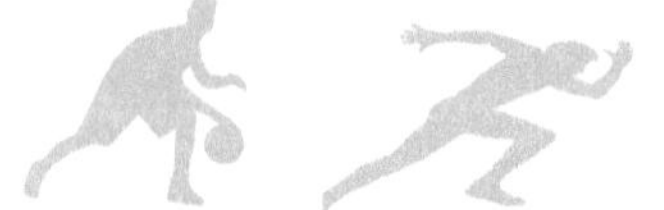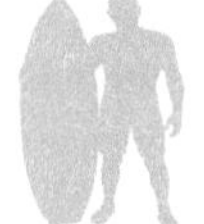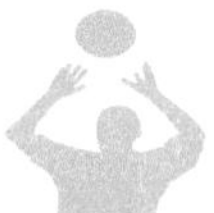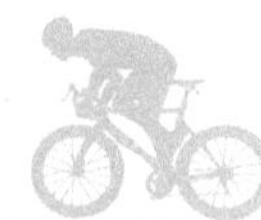

Cardio

ACTIVITY	DISTANCE	TIME	TARGET HEART RATE

Strength Training

EXERCISE	SET ONE WEIGHT/REPS	SET TWO WEIGHT/REPS	SET THREE WEIGHT/REPS

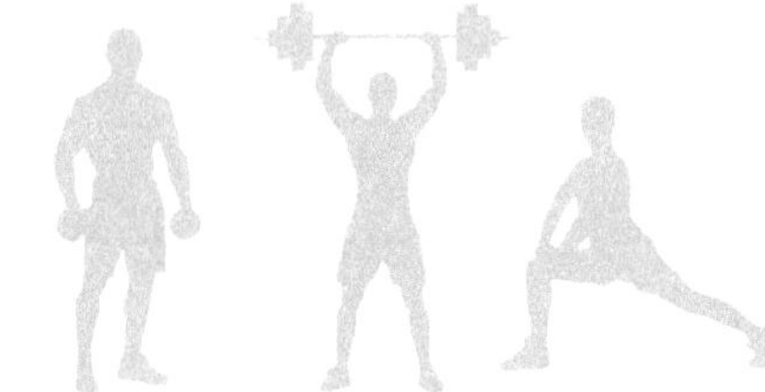

Name: ....

Date: ....

Time: ....

Warm-Up

ACTIVITY	TIME	REPS

Cardio

ACTIVITY	DISTANCE	TIME	TARGET HEART RATE

Strength Training

EXERCISE	SET ONE WEIGHT/REPS	SET TWO WEIGHT/REPS	SET THREE WEIGHT/REPS

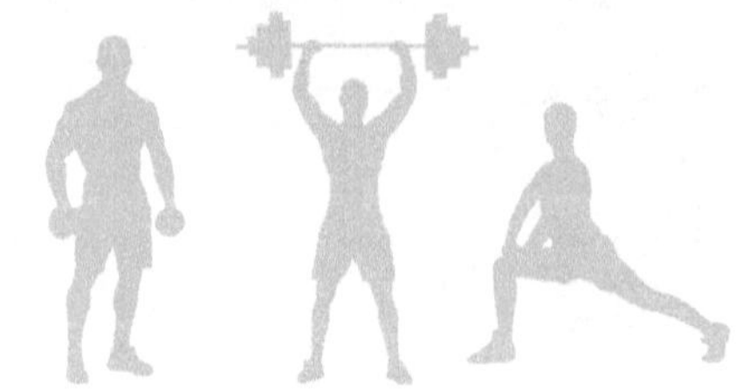

Name: ....

Date: ....

Time: ....

Warm-Up

ACTIVITY	TIME	REPS

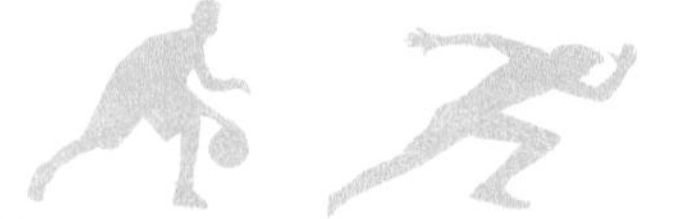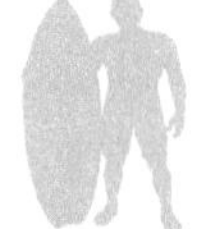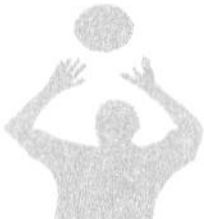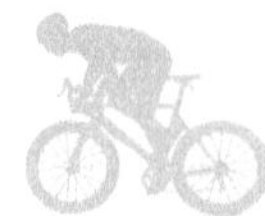

Cardio

ACTIVITY	DISTANCE	TIME	TARGET HEART RATE

Strength Training

EXERCISE	SET ONE WEIGHT/REPS	SET TWO WEIGHT/REPS	SET THREE WEIGHT/REPS

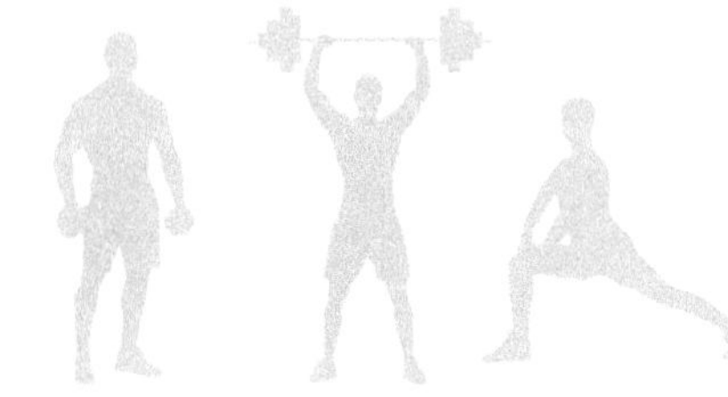

Warm-Up

ACTIVITY	TIME	REPS

Cardio

ACTIVITY	DISTANCE	TIME	TARGET HEART RATE

Strength Training

EXERCISE	SET ONE WEIGHT/REPS	SET TWO WEIGHT/REPS	SET THREE WEIGHT/REPS

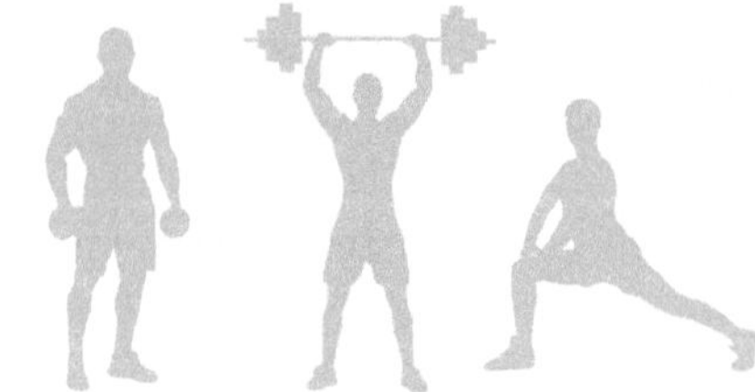

Name: ....

Date: ....

Time: ....

Warm-Up

ACTIVITY	TIME	REPS

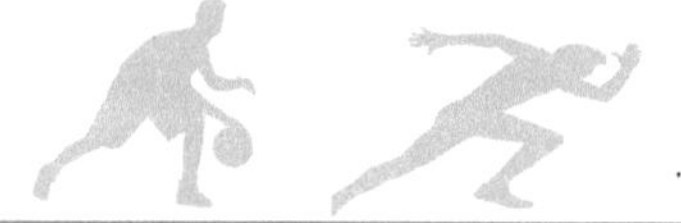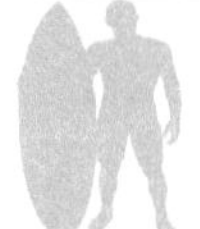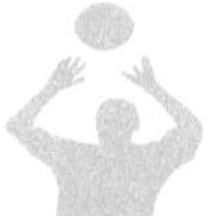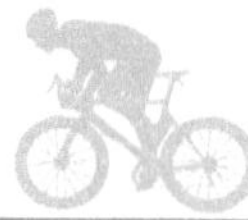

Cardio

ACTIVITY	DISTANCE	TIME	TARGET HEART RATE

Strength Training

EXERCISE	SET ONE WEIGHT/REPS	SET TWO WEIGHT/REPS	SET THREE WEIGHT/REPS

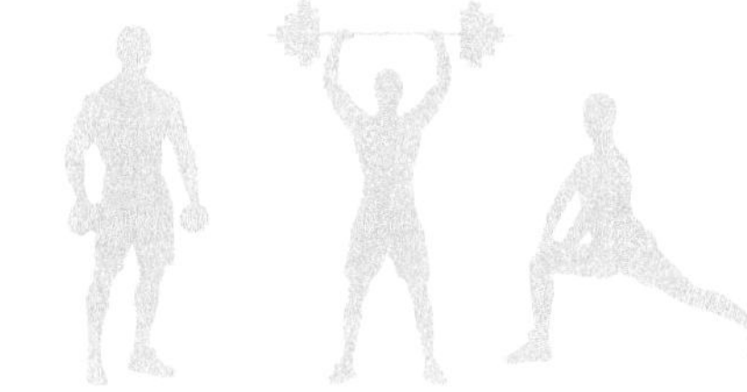

Warm-Up

ACTIVITY	TIME	REPS

Cardio

ACTIVITY	DISTANCE	TIME	TARGET HEART RATE

Strength Training

EXERCISE	SET ONE WEIGHT/REPS	SET TWO WEIGHT/REPS	SET THREE WEIGHT/REPS

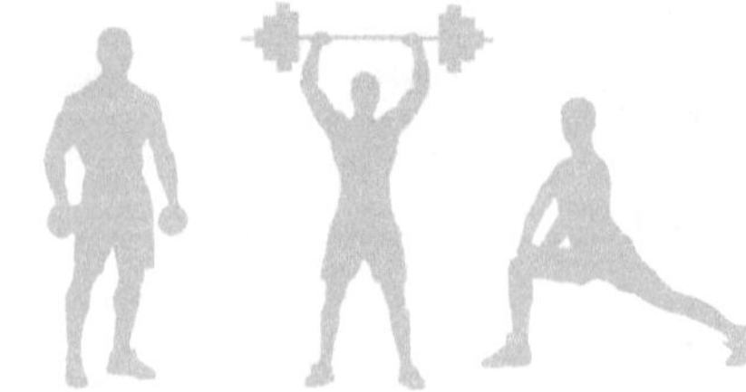

Name: ....

Date: ....

Time: ....

Warm-Up

ACTIVITY	TIME	REPS

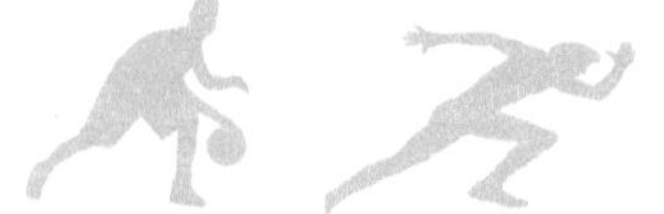 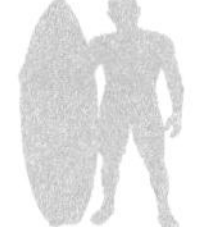 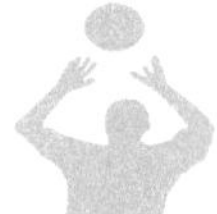 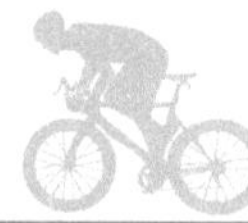

Cardio

ACTIVITY	DISTANCE	TIME	TARGET HEART RATE

Strength Training

EXERCISE	SET ONE WEIGHT/REPS	SET TWO WEIGHT/REPS	SET THREE WEIGHT/REPS

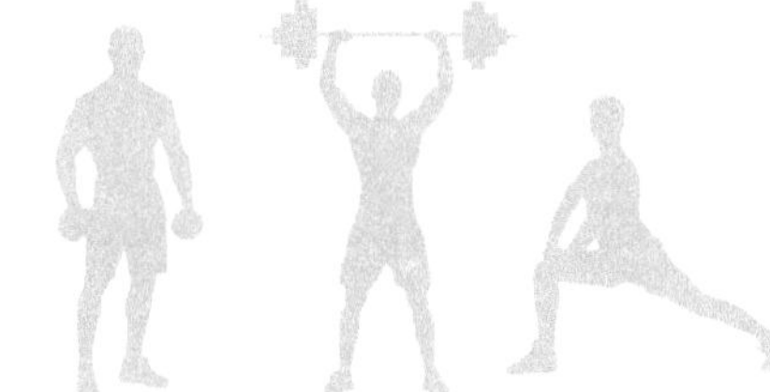

Name: ....

Date: ....

Time: ....

Warm-Up

ACTIVITY	TIME	REPS

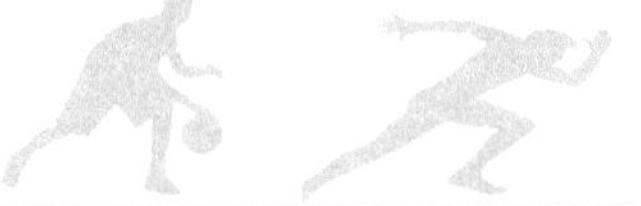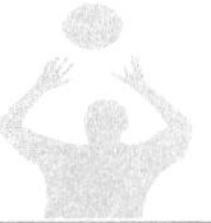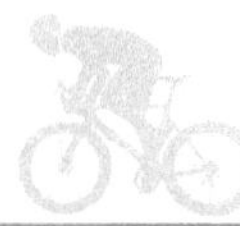

Cardio

ACTIVITY	DISTANCE	TIME	TARGET HEART RATE

Strength Training

EXERCISE	SET ONE WEIGHT/REPS	SET TWO WEIGHT/REPS	SET THREE WEIGHT/REPS

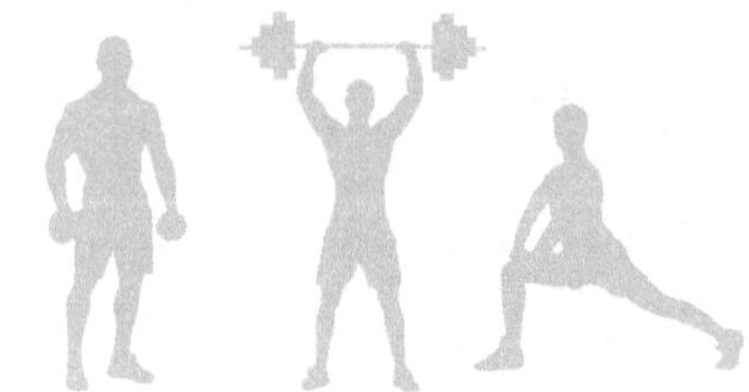

Name: ....

Date: ....

Time: ....

Warm-Up

ACTIVITY	TIME	REPS

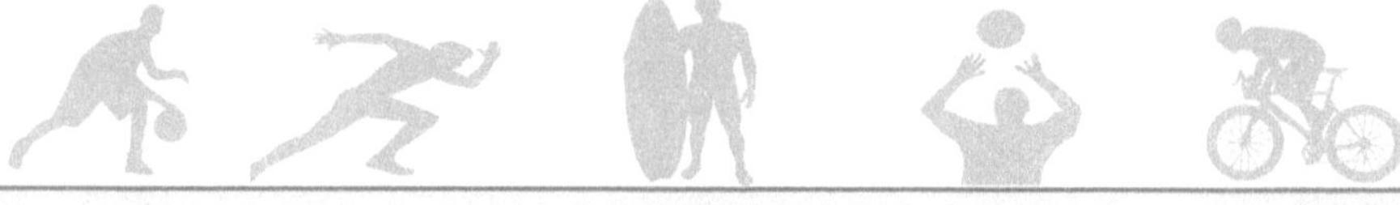

Cardio

ACTIVITY	DISTANCE	TIME	TARGET HEART RATE

Strength Training

EXERCISE	SET ONE WEIGHT/REPS	SET TWO WEIGHT/REPS	SET THREE WEIGHT/REPS

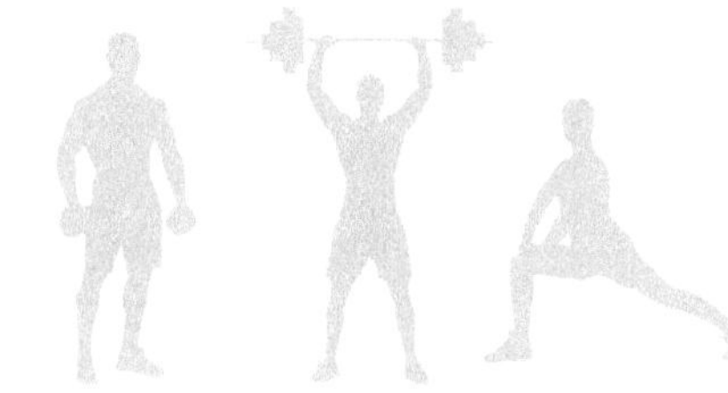

Name: ....

Date: ....

Time: ....

Warm-Up

ACTIVITY	TIME	REPS

Cardio

ACTIVITY	DISTANCE	TIME	TARGET HEART RATE

Strength Training

EXERCISE	SET ONE WEIGHT/REPS	SET TWO WEIGHT/REPS	SET THREE WEIGHT/REPS

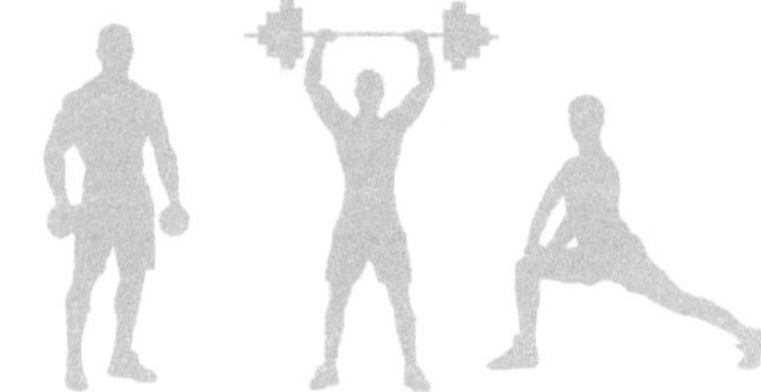

Name: ....

Date: ....

Time: ....

Warm-Up

ACTIVITY	TIME	REPS

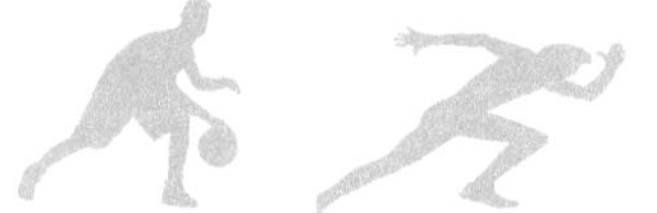 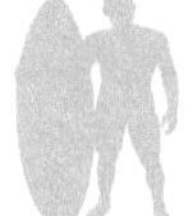 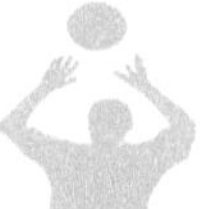 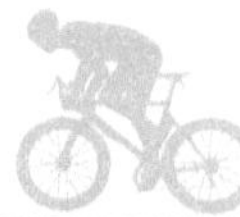

Cardio

ACTIVITY	DISTANCE	TIME	TARGET HEART RATE

Strength Training

EXERCISE	SET ONE WEIGHT/REPS	SET TWO WEIGHT/REPS	SET THREE WEIGHT/REPS

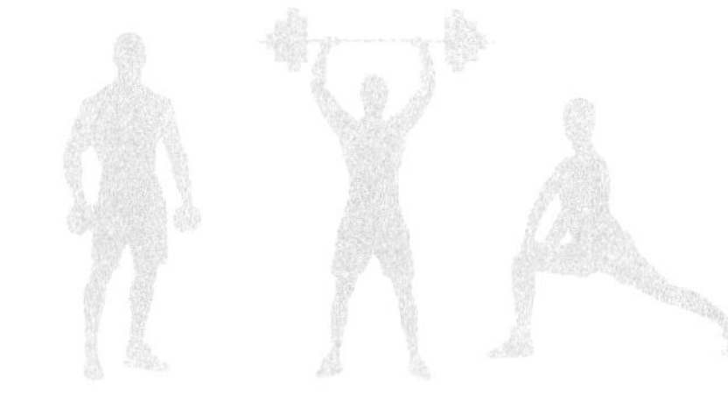

Name: ....

Date: ....

Time: ....

Warm-Up

ACTIVITY	TIME	REPS

Cardio

ACTIVITY	DISTANCE	TIME	TARGET HEART RATE

Strength Training

EXERCISE	SET ONE WEIGHT/REPS	SET TWO WEIGHT/REPS	SET THREE WEIGHT/REPS

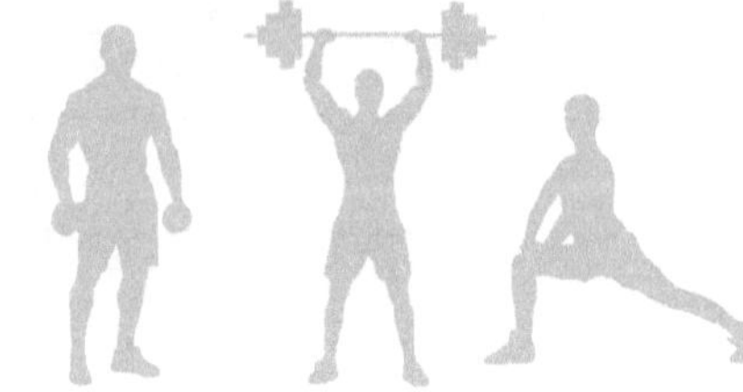

Name: ....

Date: ....

Time: ....

Warm-Up

ACTIVITY	TIME	REPS

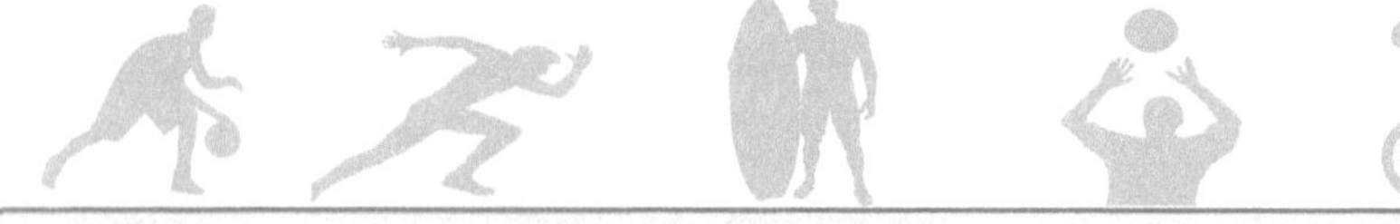

Cardio

ACTIVITY	DISTANCE	TIME	TARGET HEART RATE

Strength Training

EXERCISE	SET ONE WEIGHT/REPS	SET TWO WEIGHT/REPS	SET THREE WEIGHT/REPS

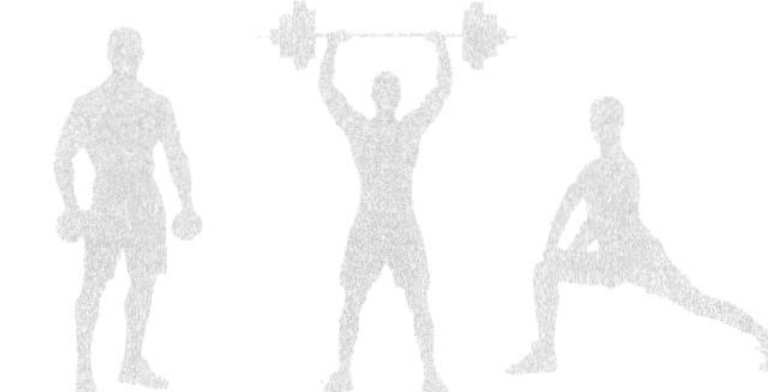

Name: ....

Date: ....

Time: ....

Warm-Up

ACTIVITY	TIME	REPS

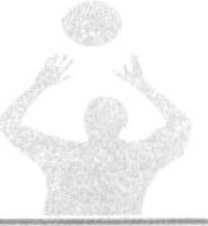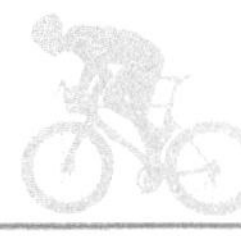

Cardio

ACTIVITY	DISTANCE	TIME	TARGET HEART RATE

Strength Training

EXERCISE	SET ONE WEIGHT/REPS	SET TWO WEIGHT/REPS	SET THREE WEIGHT/REPS

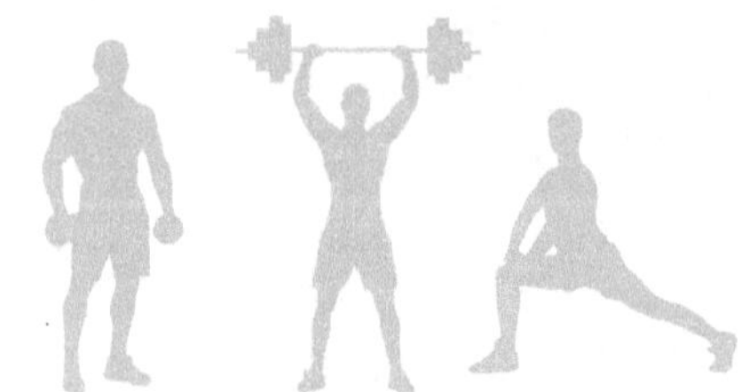

Name: ....

Date: ....

Time: ....

Warm-Up

ACTIVITY	TIME	REPS

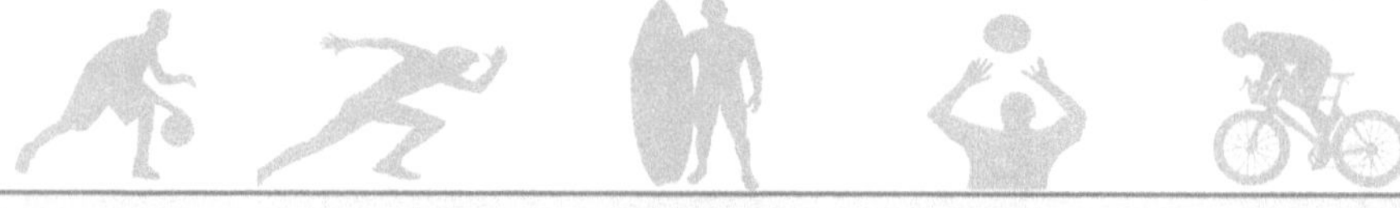

Cardio

ACTIVITY	DISTANCE	TIME	TARGET HEART RATE

Strength Training

EXERCISE	SET ONE WEIGHT/REPS	SET TWO WEIGHT/REPS	SET THREE WEIGHT/REPS

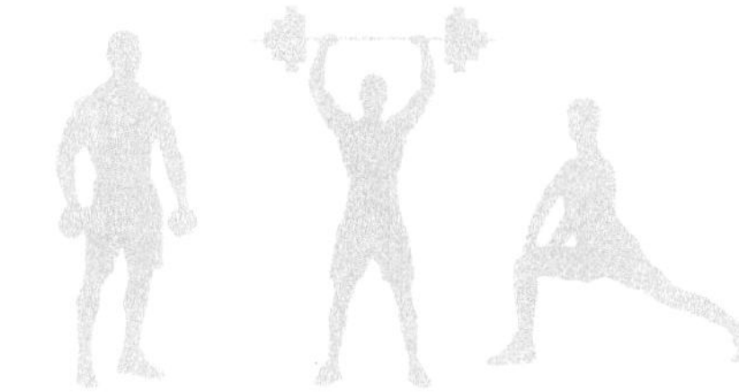

Name: ....

Date: ....

Time: ....

Warm-Up

ACTIVITY	TIME	REPS

Cardio

ACTIVITY	DISTANCE	TIME	TARGET HEART RATE

Strength Training

EXERCISE	SET ONE WEIGHT/REPS	SET TWO WEIGHT/REPS	SET THREE WEIGHT/REPS

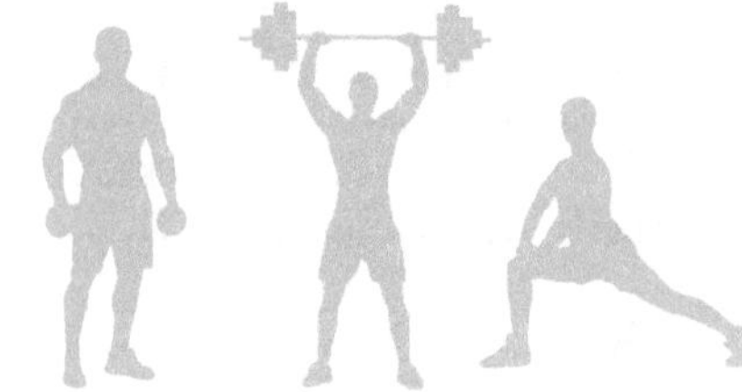

Name: ....

Date: ....

Time: ....

Warm-Up

ACTIVITY	TIME	REPS

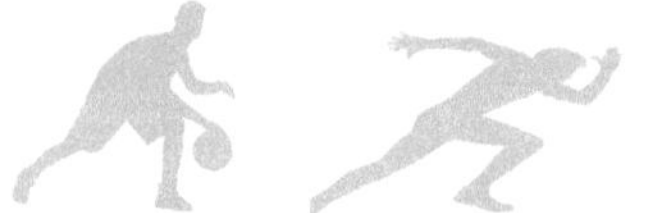 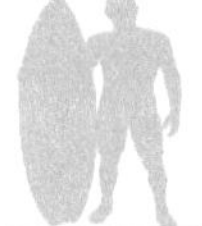 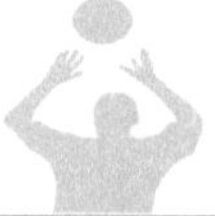 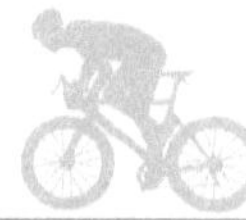

Cardio

ACTIVITY	DISTANCE	TIME	TARGET HEART RATE

Strength Training

EXERCISE	SET ONE WEIGHT/REPS	SET TWO WEIGHT/REPS	SET THREE WEIGHT/REPS

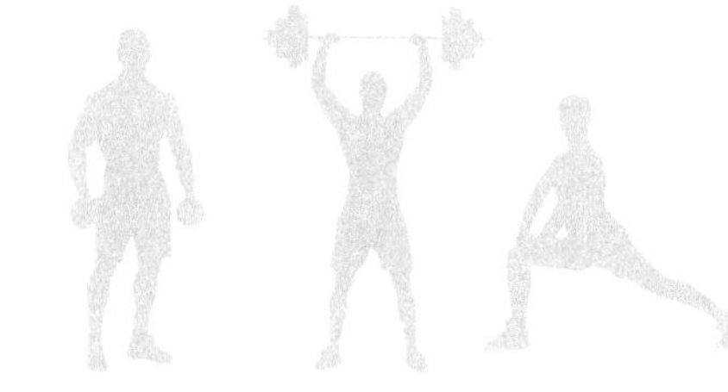

Name: ....

Date: ....

Time: ....

Warm-Up

ACTIVITY	TIME	REPS

Cardio

ACTIVITY	DISTANCE	TIME	TARGET HEART RATE

Strength Training

EXERCISE	SET ONE WEIGHT/REPS	SET TWO WEIGHT/REPS	SET THREE WEIGHT/REPS

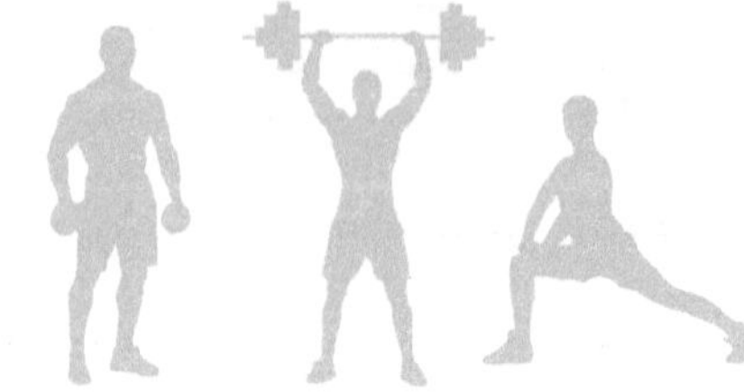

Name: ....

Date: ....

Time: ....

Warm-Up

ACTIVITY	TIME	REPS

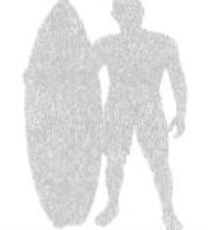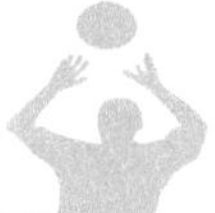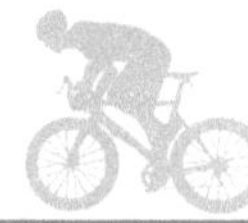

Cardio

ACTIVITY	DISTANCE	TIME	TARGET HEART RATE

Strength Training

EXERCISE	SET ONE WEIGHT/REPS	SET TWO WEIGHT/REPS	SET THREE WEIGHT/REPS

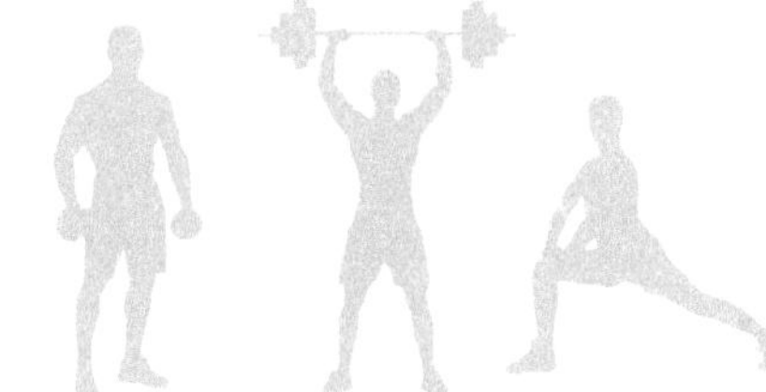

Name: ....

Date: ....

Time: ....

Warm-Up

ACTIVITY	TIME	REPS

Cardio

ACTIVITY	DISTANCE	TIME	TARGET HEART RATE

Strength Training

EXERCISE	SET ONE WEIGHT/REPS	SET TWO WEIGHT/REPS	SET THREE WEIGHT/REPS

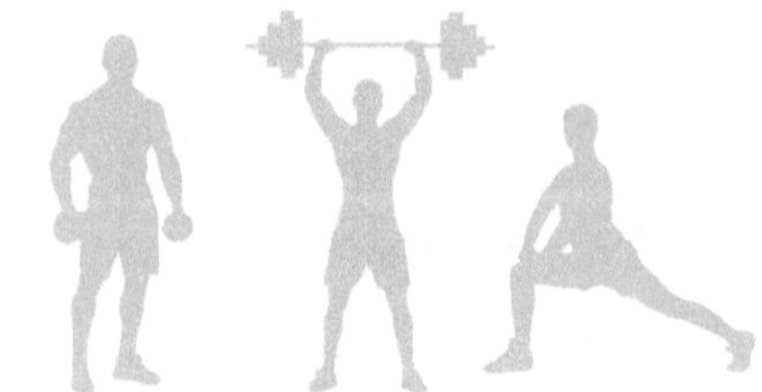

Name: ....

Date: ....

Time: ....

Warm-Up

ACTIVITY	TIME	REPS

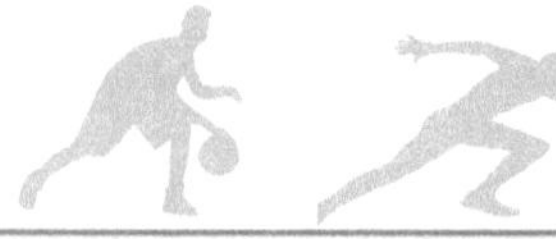 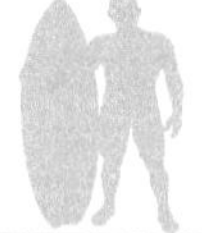 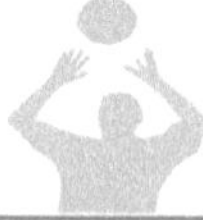 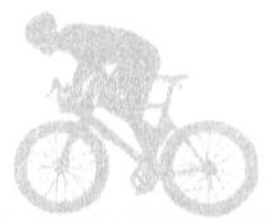

Cardio

ACTIVITY	DISTANCE	TIME	TARGET HEART RATE

Strength Training

EXERCISE	SET ONE WEIGHT/REPS	SET TWO WEIGHT/REPS	SET THREE WEIGHT/REPS

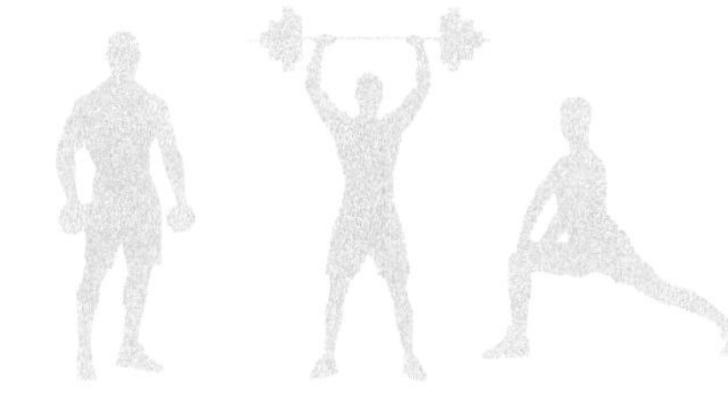

Name: ....

Date: ....

Time: ....

Warm-Up

ACTIVITY	TIME	REPS

Cardio

ACTIVITY	DISTANCE	TIME	TARGET HEART RATE

Strength Training

EXERCISE	SET ONE WEIGHT/REPS	SET TWO WEIGHT/REPS	SET THREE WEIGHT/REPS

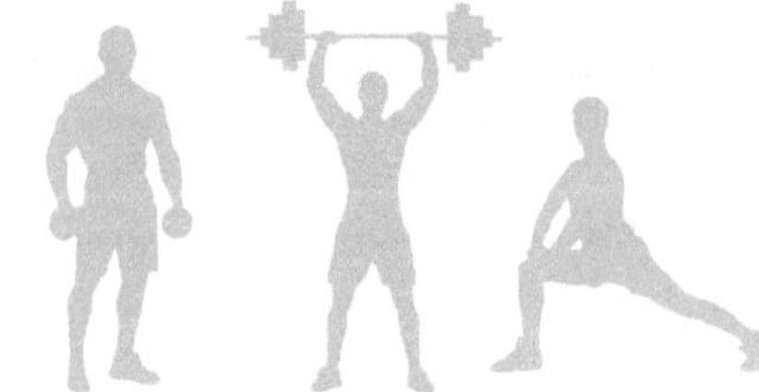

Name: ....

Date: ....

Time: ....

Warm-Up

ACTIVITY	TIME	REPS

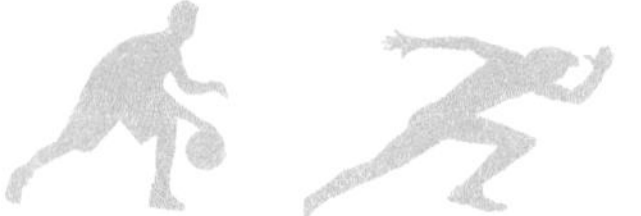 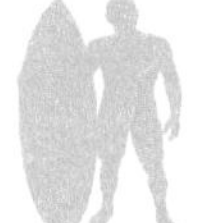 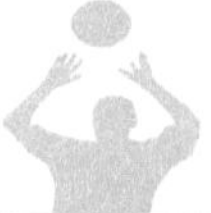 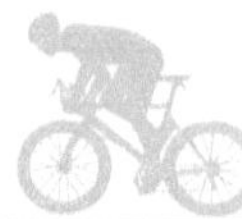

Cardio

ACTIVITY	DISTANCE	TIME	TARGET HEART RATE

Strength Training

EXERCISE	SET ONE WEIGHT/REPS	SET TWO WEIGHT/REPS	SET THREE WEIGHT/REPS

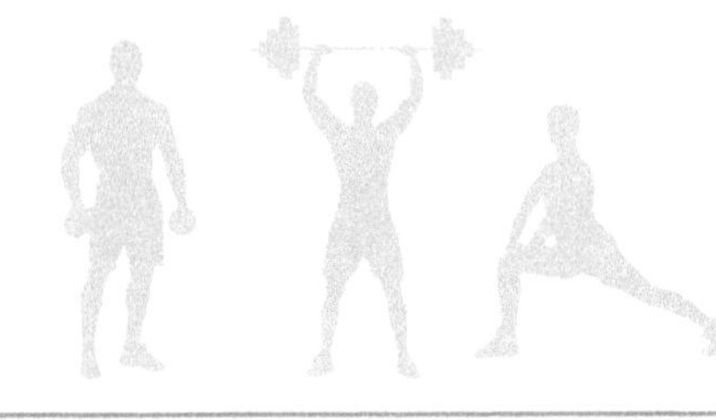

Warm-Up

ACTIVITY	TIME	REPS

Cardio

ACTIVITY	DISTANCE	TIME	TARGET HEART RATE

Strength Training

EXERCISE	SET ONE WEIGHT/REPS	SET TWO WEIGHT/REPS	SET THREE WEIGHT/REPS

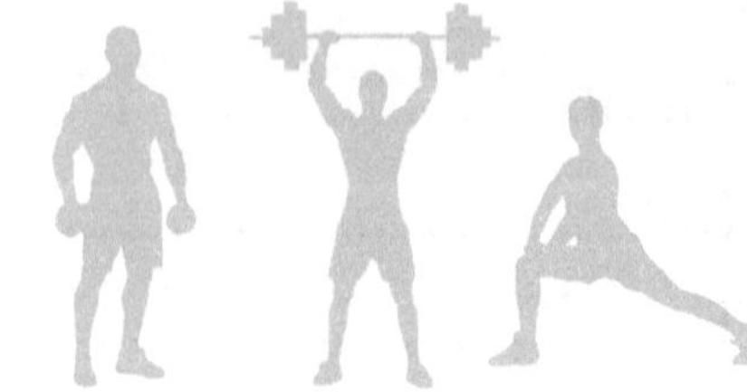

Name: ....

Date: ....

Time: ....

Warm-Up

ACTIVITY	TIME	REPS

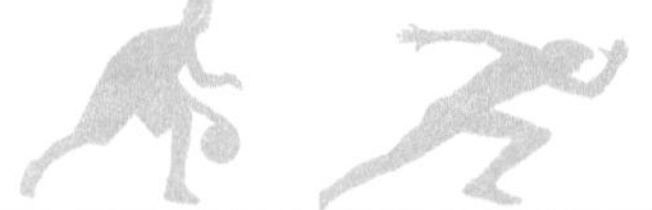 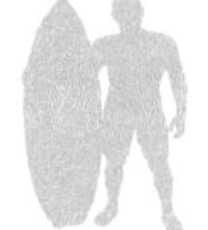 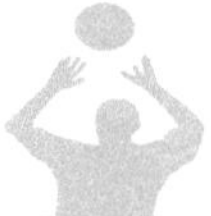 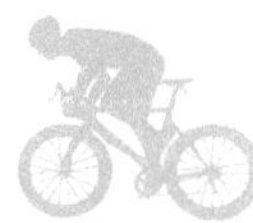

Cardio

ACTIVITY	DISTANCE	TIME	TARGET HEART RATE

Strength Training

EXERCISE	SET ONE WEIGHT/REPS	SET TWO WEIGHT/REPS	SET THREE WEIGHT/REPS

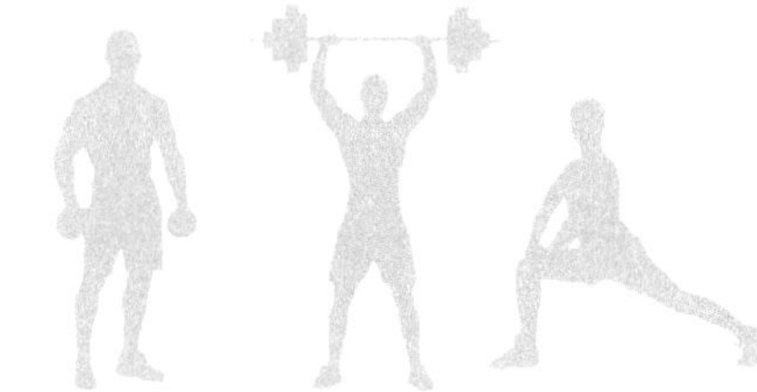

Name: ....

Date: ....

Time: ....

Warm-Up

ACTIVITY	TIME	REPS

Cardio

ACTIVITY	DISTANCE	TIME	TARGET HEART RATE

Strength Training

EXERCISE	SET ONE WEIGHT/REPS	SET TWO WEIGHT/REPS	SET THREE WEIGHT/REPS

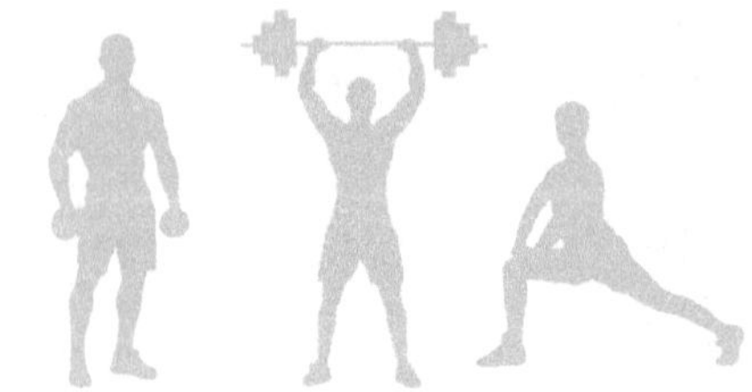

Name: ....

Date: ....

Time: ....

Warm-Up

ACTIVITY	TIME	REPS

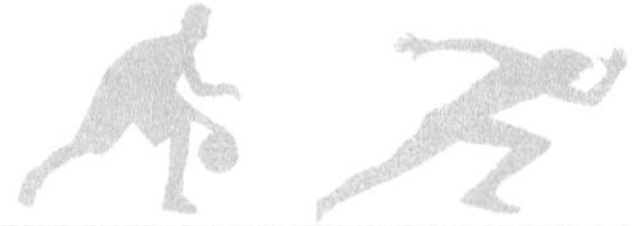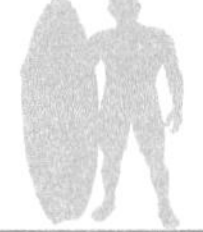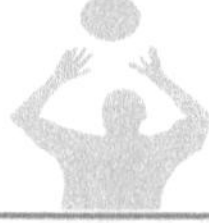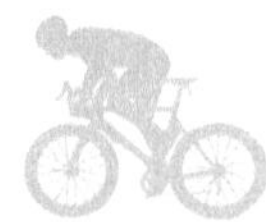

Cardio

ACTIVITY	DISTANCE	TIME	TARGET HEART RATE

Strength Training

EXERCISE	SET ONE WEIGHT/REPS	SET TWO WEIGHT/REPS	SET THREE WEIGHT/REPS

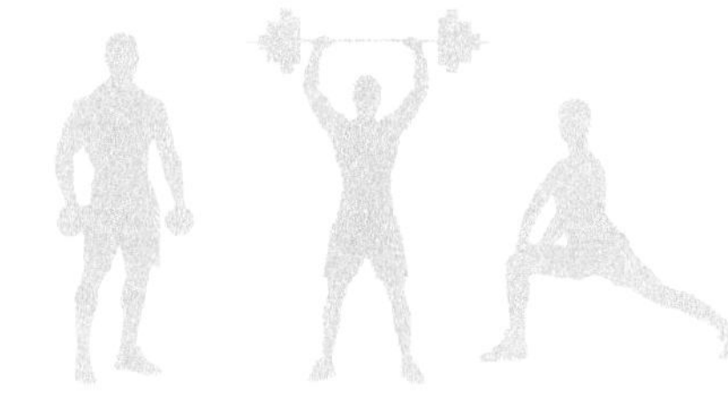

Name: ....

Date: ....

Time: ....

Warm-Up

ACTIVITY	TIME	REPS

Cardio

ACTIVITY	DISTANCE	TIME	TARGET HEART RATE

Strength Training

EXERCISE	SET ONE WEIGHT/REPS	SET TWO WEIGHT/REPS	SET THREE WEIGHT/REPS

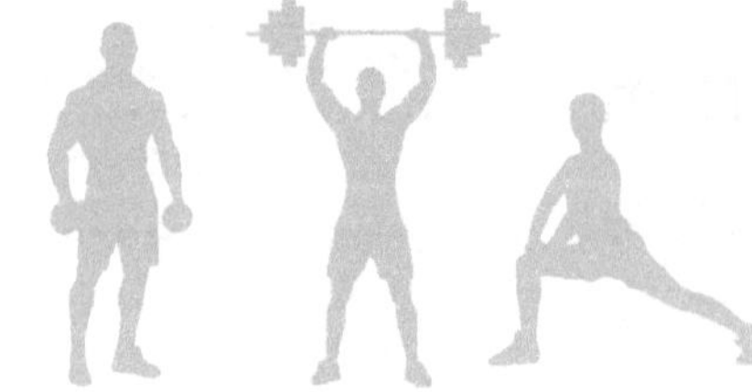

Name: ....

Date: ....

Time: ....

Warm-Up

ACTIVITY	TIME	REPS

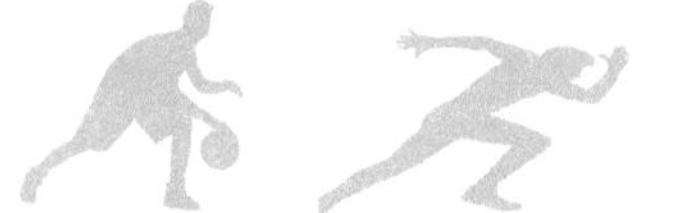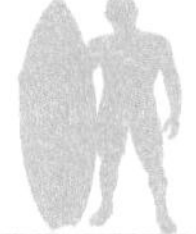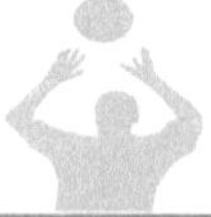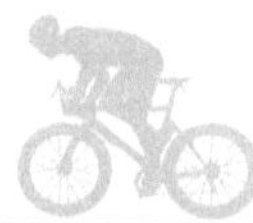

Cardio

ACTIVITY	DISTANCE	TIME	TARGET HEART RATE

Strength Training

EXERCISE	SET ONE WEIGHT/REPS	SET TWO WEIGHT/REPS	SET THREE WEIGHT/REPS

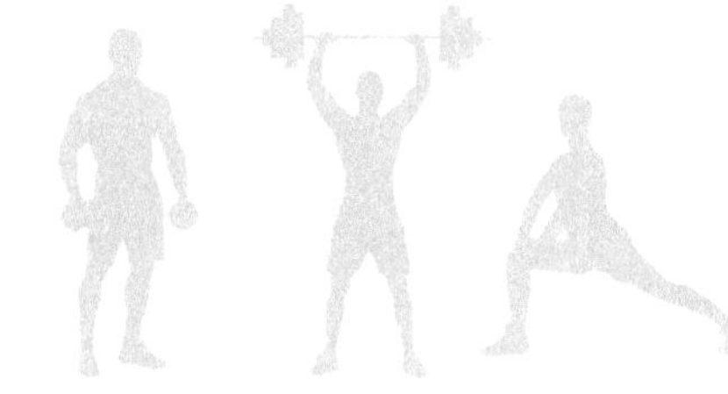

Name: ....

Date: ....

Time: ....

Warm-Up

ACTIVITY	TIME	REPS

Cardio

ACTIVITY	DISTANCE	TIME	TARGET HEART RATE

Strength Training

EXERCISE	SET ONE WEIGHT/REPS	SET TWO WEIGHT/REPS	SET THREE WEIGHT/REPS

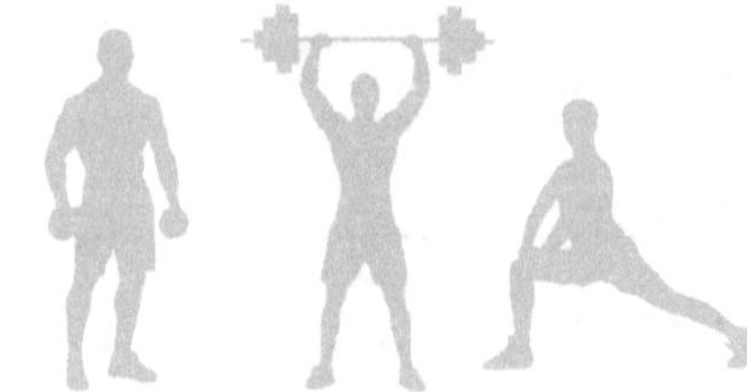

Name: ....

Date: ....

Time: ....

Warm-Up

ACTIVITY	TIME	REPS

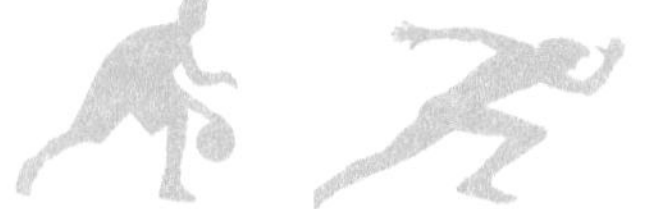 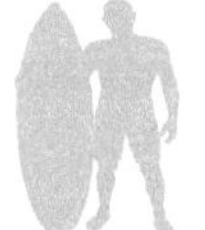 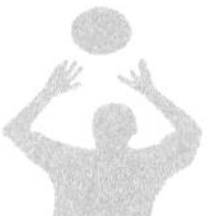 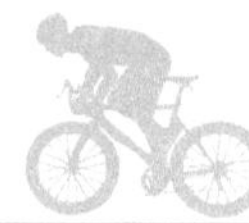

Cardio

ACTIVITY	DISTANCE	TIME	TARGET HEART RATE

Strength Training

EXERCISE	SET ONE WEIGHT/REPS	SET TWO WEIGHT/REPS	SET THREE WEIGHT/REPS

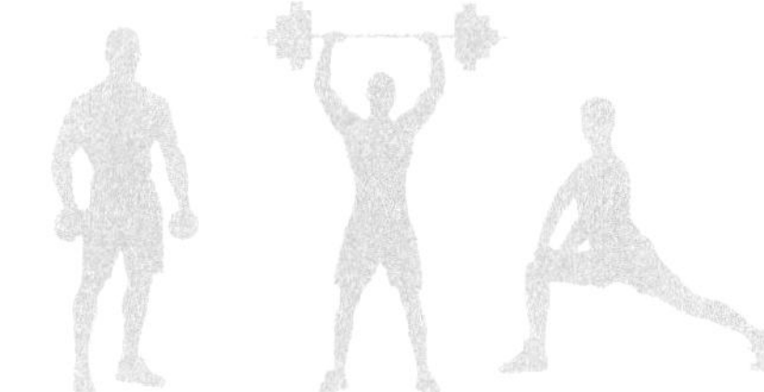

Name: ....

Date: ....

Time: ....

Warm-Up

ACTIVITY	TIME	REPS

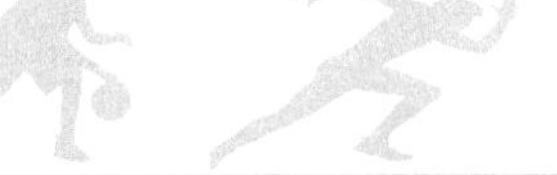 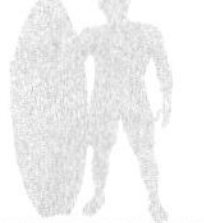 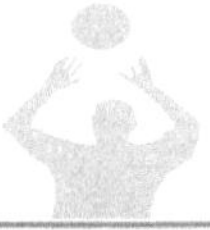 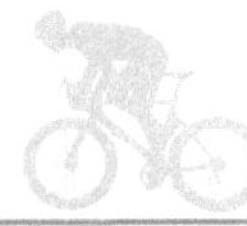

Cardio

ACTIVITY	DISTANCE	TIME	TARGET HEART RATE

Strength Training

EXERCISE	SET ONE WEIGHT/REPS	SET TWO WEIGHT/REPS	SET THREE WEIGHT/REPS

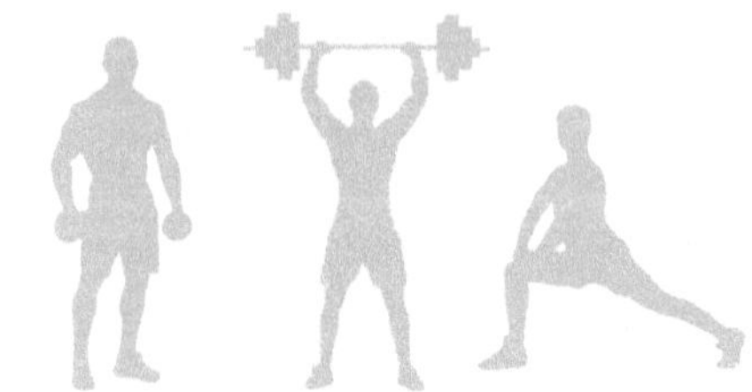

Name: ....

Date: ....

Time: ....

Warm-Up

ACTIVITY	TIME	REPS

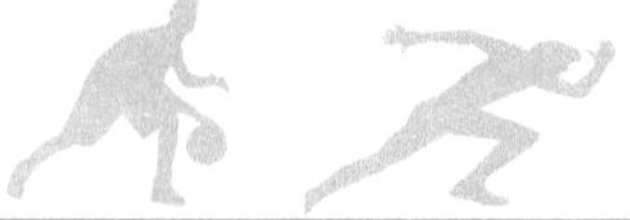 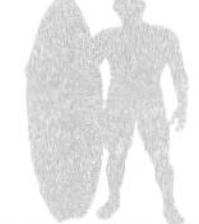 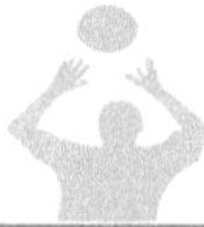 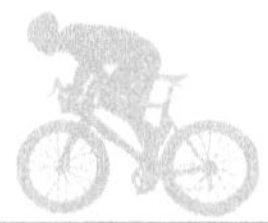

Cardio

ACTIVITY	DISTANCE	TIME	TARGET HEART RATE

Strength Training

EXERCISE	SET ONE WEIGHT/REPS	SET TWO WEIGHT/REPS	SET THREE WEIGHT/REPS

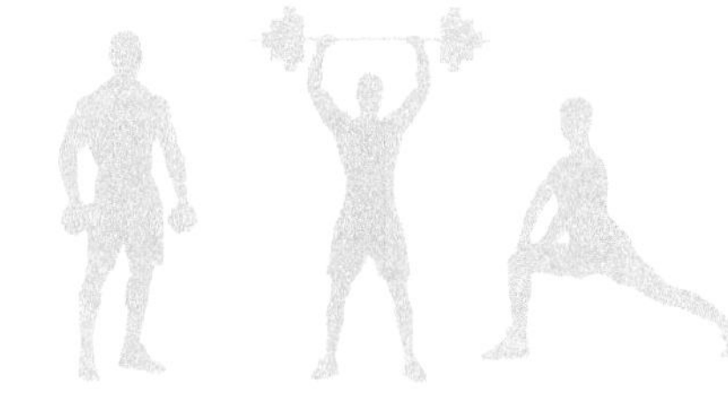

Name: ……………………….

Date: …………………………

Time: …………………………

Warm-Up

ACTIVITY	TIME	REPS

Cardio

ACTIVITY	DISTANCE	TIME	TARGET HEART RATE

Strength Training

EXERCISE	SET ONE WEIGHT/REPS	SET TWO WEIGHT/REPS	SET THREE WEIGHT/REPS

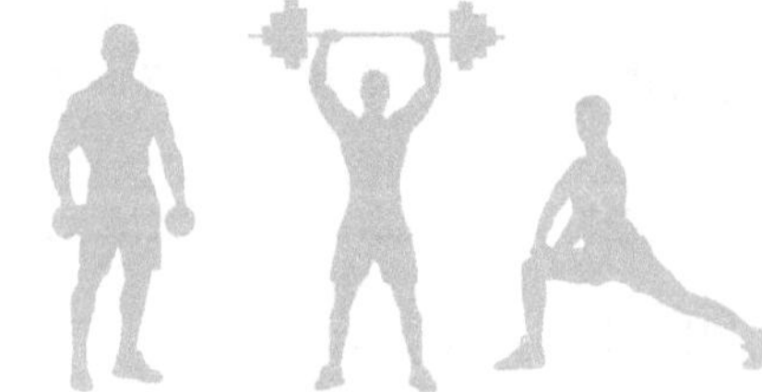

Name: ....

Date: ....

Time: ....

Warm-Up

ACTIVITY	TIME	REPS

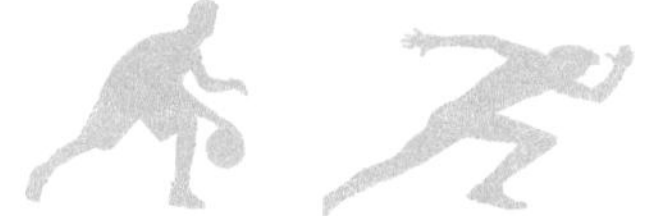 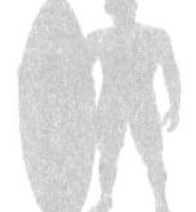 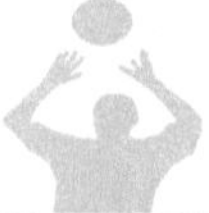 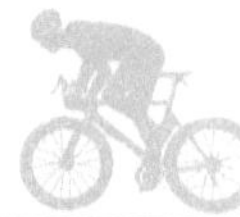

Cardio

ACTIVITY	DISTANCE	TIME	TARGET HEART RATE

Strength Training

EXERCISE	SET ONE WEIGHT/REPS	SET TWO WEIGHT/REPS	SET THREE WEIGHT/REPS

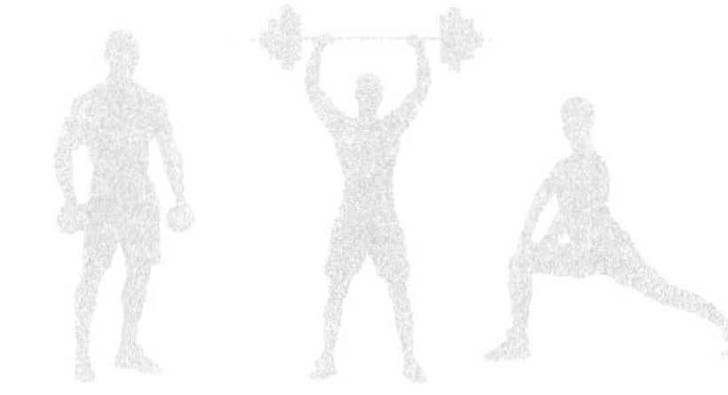

Name: ....

Date: ....

Time: ....

Warm-Up

ACTIVITY	TIME	REPS

Cardio

ACTIVITY	DISTANCE	TIME	TARGET HEART RATE

Strength Training

EXERCISE	SET ONE WEIGHT/REPS	SET TWO WEIGHT/REPS	SET THREE WEIGHT/REPS

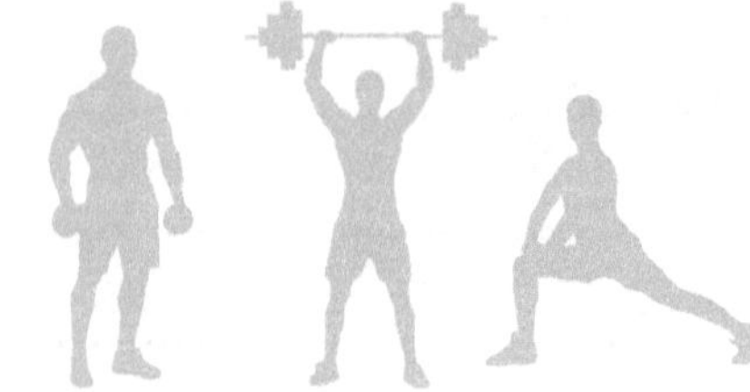

Name: ....

Date: ....

Time: ....

Warm-Up

ACTIVITY	TIME	REPS

 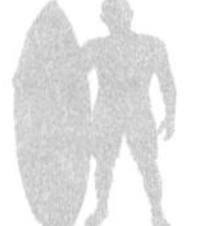 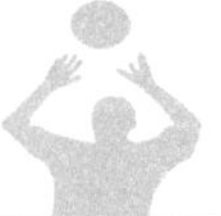 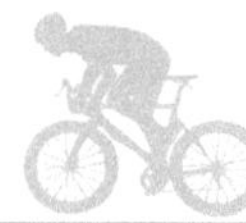

Cardio

ACTIVITY	DISTANCE	TIME	TARGET HEART RATE

Strength Training

EXERCISE	SET ONE WEIGHT/REPS	SET TWO WEIGHT/REPS	SET THREE WEIGHT/REPS

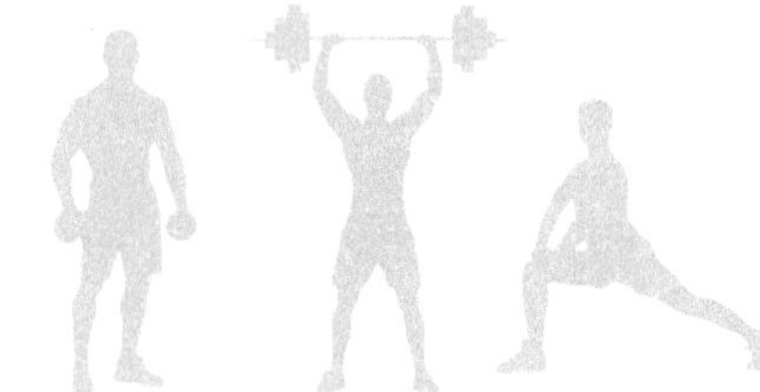

Name: ....

Date: ....

Time: ....

Warm-Up

ACTIVITY	TIME	REPS

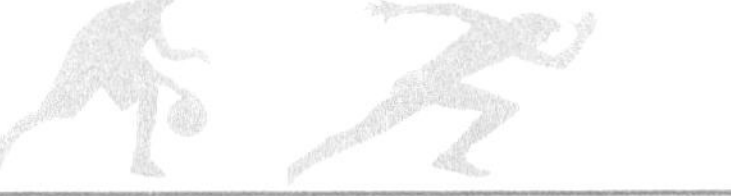  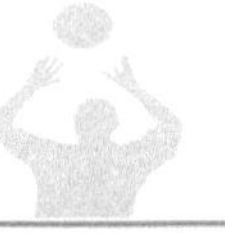 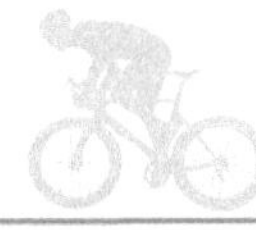

Cardio

ACTIVITY	DISTANCE	TIME	TARGET HEART RATE

Strength Training

EXERCISE	SET ONE WEIGHT/REPS	SET TWO WEIGHT/REPS	SET THREE WEIGHT/REPS

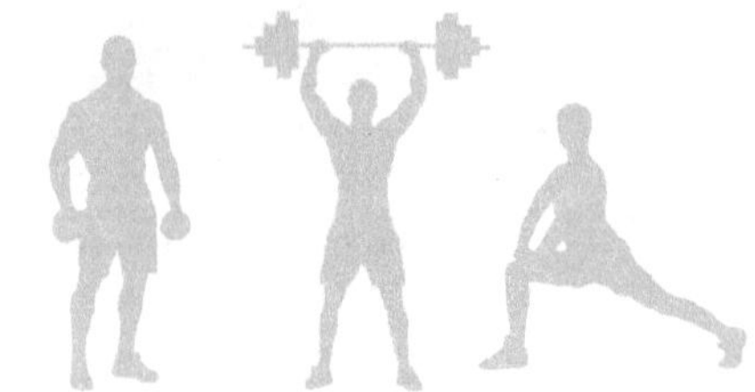

Name: ....

Date: ....

Time: ....

Warm-Up

ACTIVITY	TIME	REPS

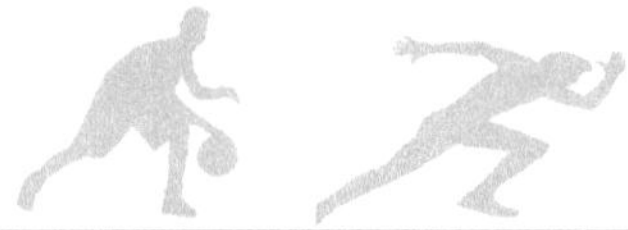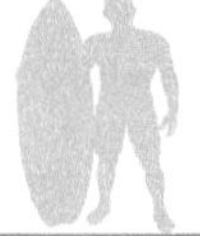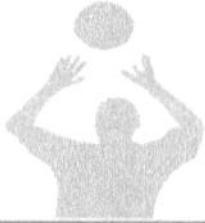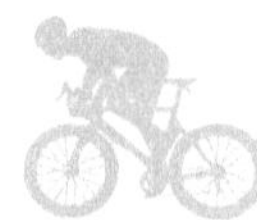

Cardio

ACTIVITY	DISTANCE	TIME	TARGET HEART RATE

Strength Training

EXERCISE	SET ONE WEIGHT/REPS	SET TWO WEIGHT/REPS	SET THREE WEIGHT/REPS

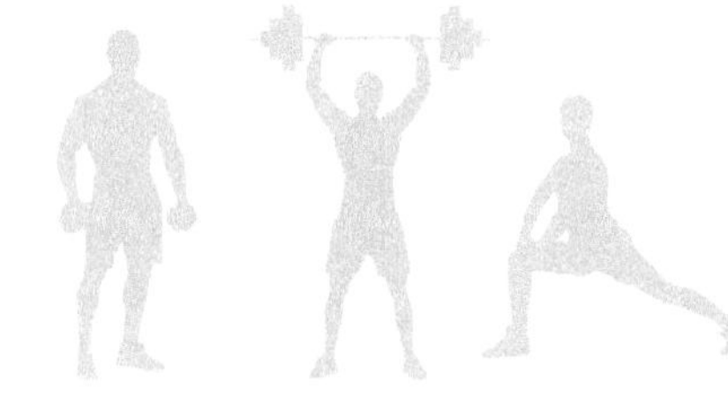

Name: ……………………………..

Date: ……………………………..

Time: ……………………………..

Warm-Up

ACTIVITY	TIME	REPS

Cardio

ACTIVITY	DISTANCE	TIME	TARGET HEART RATE

Strength Training

EXERCISE	SET ONE WEIGHT/REPS	SET TWO WEIGHT/REPS	SET THREE WEIGHT/REPS

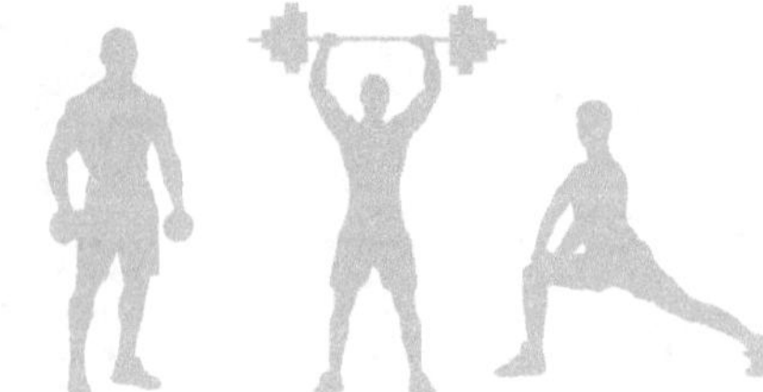

Name: ....

Date: ....

Time: ....

Warm-Up

ACTIVITY	TIME	REPS

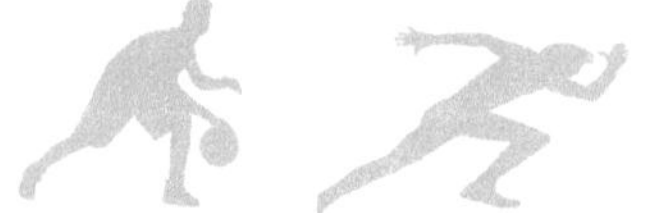 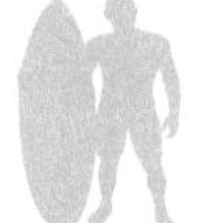 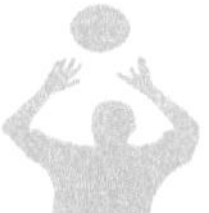 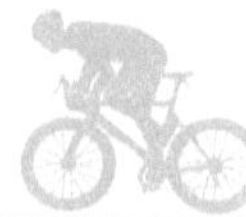

Cardio

ACTIVITY	DISTANCE	TIME	TARGET HEART RATE

Strength Training

EXERCISE	SET ONE WEIGHT/REPS	SET TWO WEIGHT/REPS	SET THREE WEIGHT/REPS

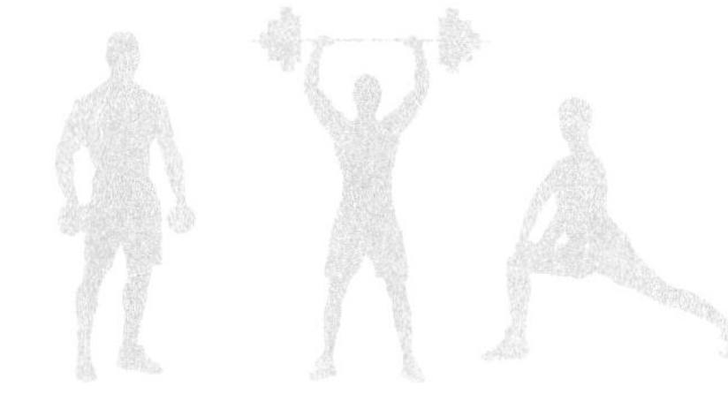

Name: ....

Date: ....

Time: ....

Warm-Up

ACTIVITY	TIME	REPS

Cardio

ACTIVITY	DISTANCE	TIME	TARGET HEART RATE

Strength Training

EXERCISE	SET ONE WEIGHT/REPS	SET TWO WEIGHT/REPS	SET THREE WEIGHT/REPS

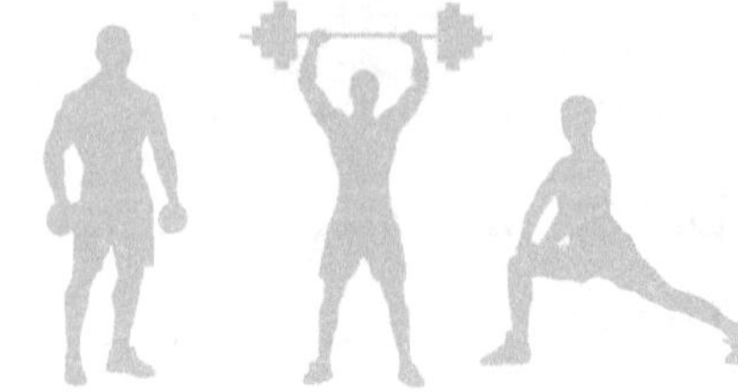

Name: ....

Date: ....

Time: ....

Warm-Up

ACTIVITY	TIME	REPS

 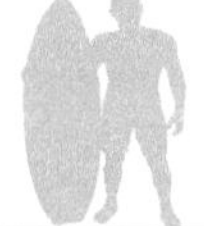 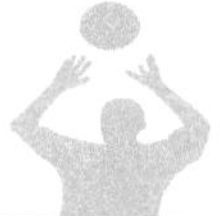 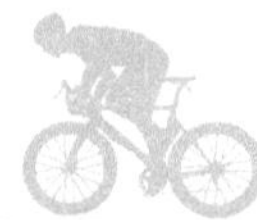

Cardio

ACTIVITY	DISTANCE	TIME	TARGET HEART RATE

Strength Training

EXERCISE	SET ONE WEIGHT/REPS	SET TWO WEIGHT/REPS	SET THREE WEIGHT/REPS

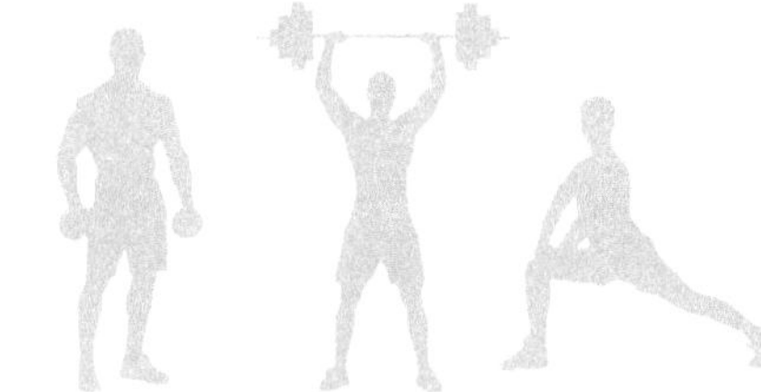

Name: ....

Date: ....

Time: ....

Warm-Up

ACTIVITY	TIME	REPS

 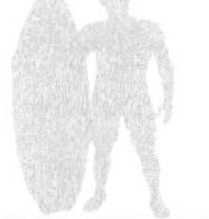 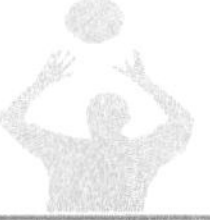 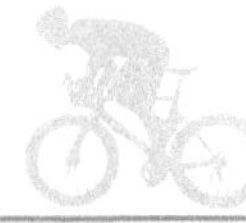

Cardio

ACTIVITY	DISTANCE	TIME	TARGET HEART RATE

Strength Training

EXERCISE	SET ONE WEIGHT/REPS	SET TWO WEIGHT/REPS	SET THREE WEIGHT/REPS

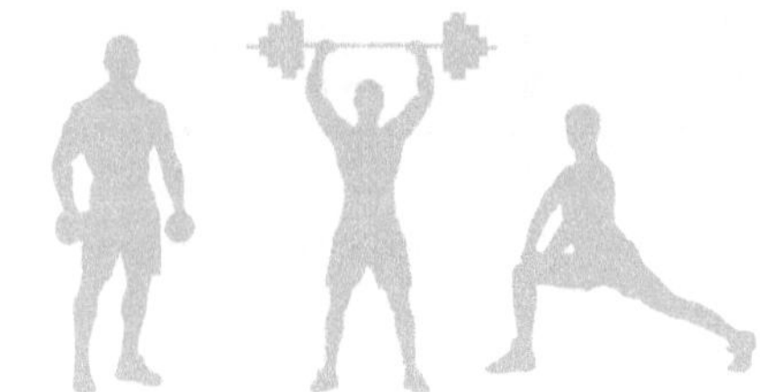

Name: ....

Date: ....

Time: ....

Warm-Up

ACTIVITY	TIME	REPS

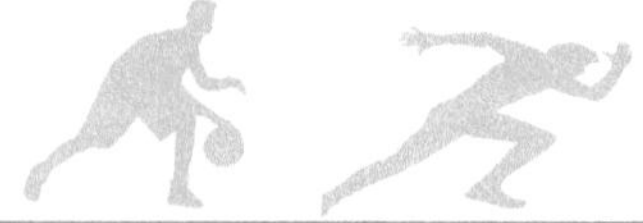 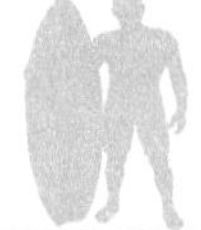 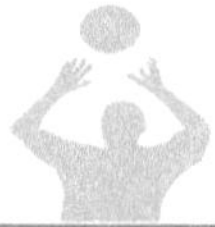 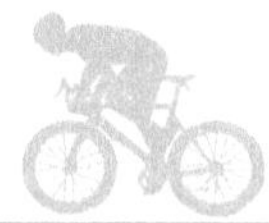

Cardio

ACTIVITY	DISTANCE	TIME	TARGET HEART RATE

Strength Training

EXERCISE	SET ONE WEIGHT/REPS	SET TWO WEIGHT/REPS	SET THREE WEIGHT/REPS

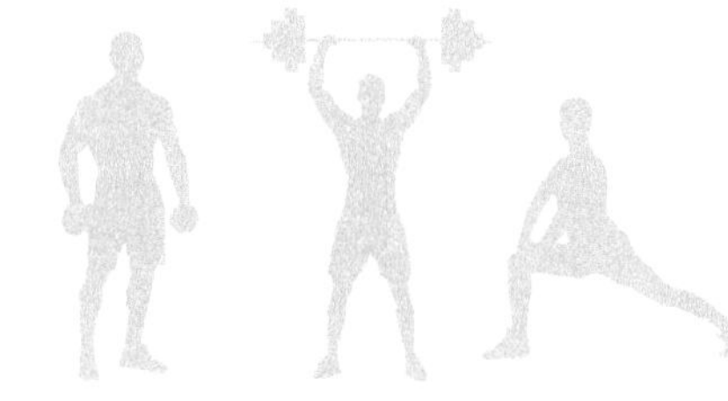

Name: ....

Date: ....

Time: ....

Warm-Up

ACTIVITY	TIME	REPS

Cardio

ACTIVITY	DISTANCE	TIME	TARGET HEART RATE

Strength Training

EXERCISE	SET ONE WEIGHT/REPS	SET TWO WEIGHT/REPS	SET THREE WEIGHT/REPS

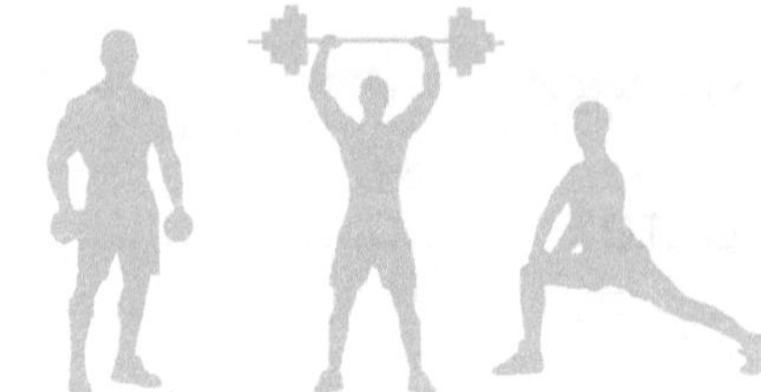

Name: ....

Date: ....

Time: ....

Warm-Up

ACTIVITY	TIME	REPS

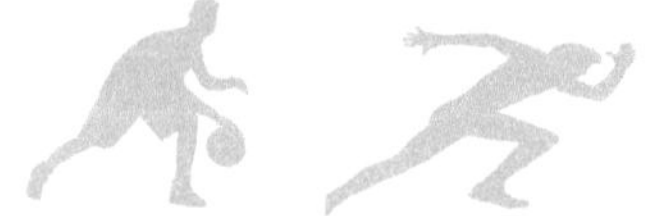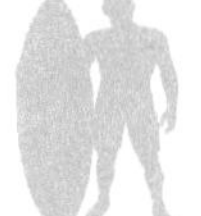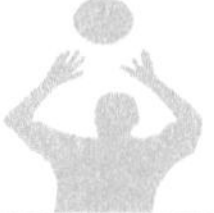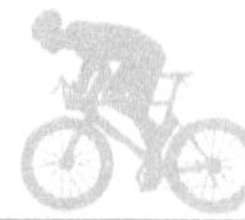

Cardio

ACTIVITY	DISTANCE	TIME	TARGET HEART RATE

Strength Training

EXERCISE	SET ONE WEIGHT/REPS	SET TWO WEIGHT/REPS	SET THREE WEIGHT/REPS

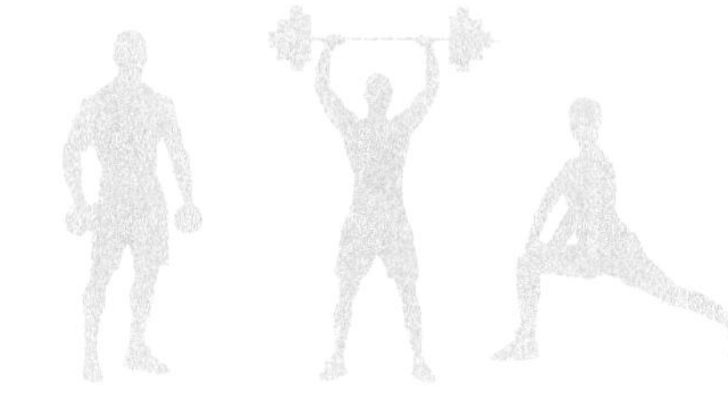

Name: ....

Date: ....

Time: ....

Warm-Up

ACTIVITY	TIME	REPS

Cardio

ACTIVITY	DISTANCE	TIME	TARGET HEART RATE

Strength Training

EXERCISE	SET ONE WEIGHT/REPS	SET TWO WEIGHT/REPS	SET THREE WEIGHT/REPS

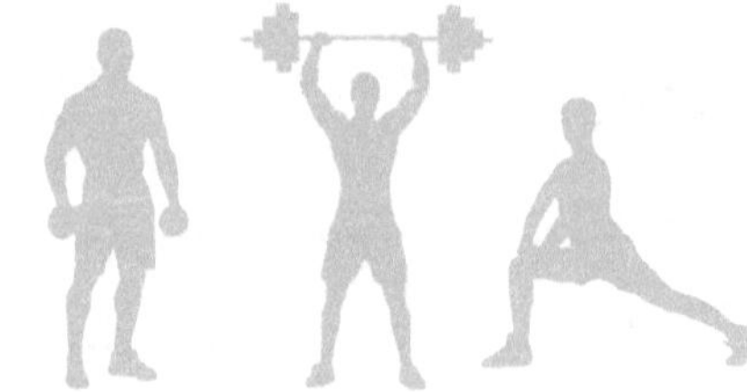

Name: ....

Date: ....

Time: ....

Warm-Up

ACTIVITY	TIME	REPS

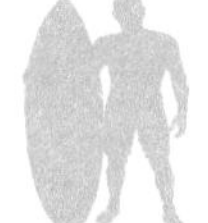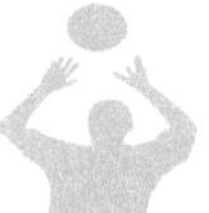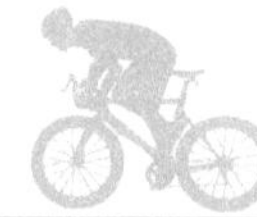

Cardio

ACTIVITY	DISTANCE	TIME	TARGET HEART RATE

Strength Training

EXERCISE	SET ONE WEIGHT/REPS	SET TWO WEIGHT/REPS	SET THREE WEIGHT/REPS

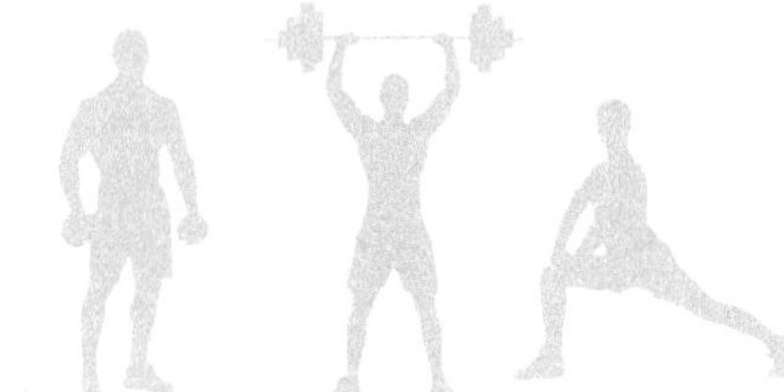

Name: ....

Date: ....

Time: ....

Warm-Up

ACTIVITY	TIME	REPS

Cardio

ACTIVITY	DISTANCE	TIME	TARGET HEART RATE

Strength Training

EXERCISE	SET ONE WEIGHT/REPS	SET TWO WEIGHT/REPS	SET THREE WEIGHT/REPS

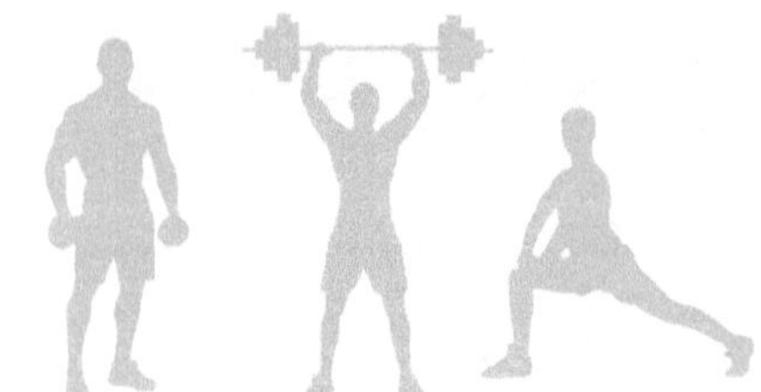

Warm-Up

ACTIVITY	TIME	REPS

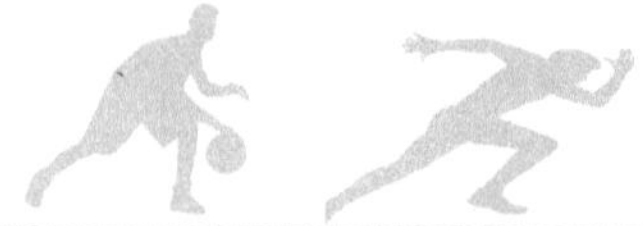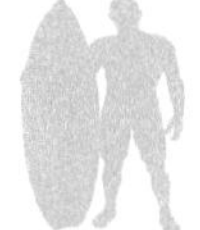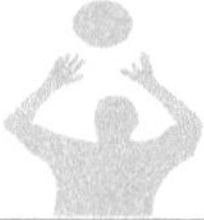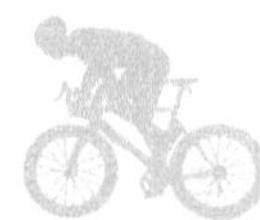

Cardio

ACTIVITY	DISTANCE	TIME	TARGET HEART RATE

Strength Training

EXERCISE	SET ONE WEIGHT/REPS	SET TWO WEIGHT/REPS	SET THREE WEIGHT/REPS

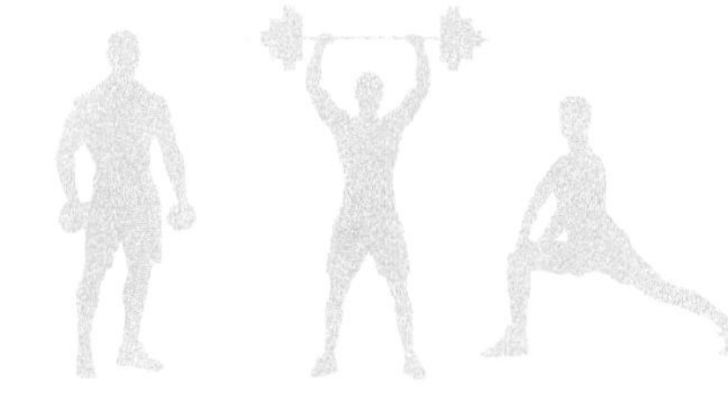

Name: ....

Date: ....

Time: ....

Warm-Up

ACTIVITY	TIME	REPS

Cardio

ACTIVITY	DISTANCE	TIME	TARGET HEART RATE

Strength Training

EXERCISE	SET ONE WEIGHT/REPS	SET TWO WEIGHT/REPS	SET THREE WEIGHT/REPS

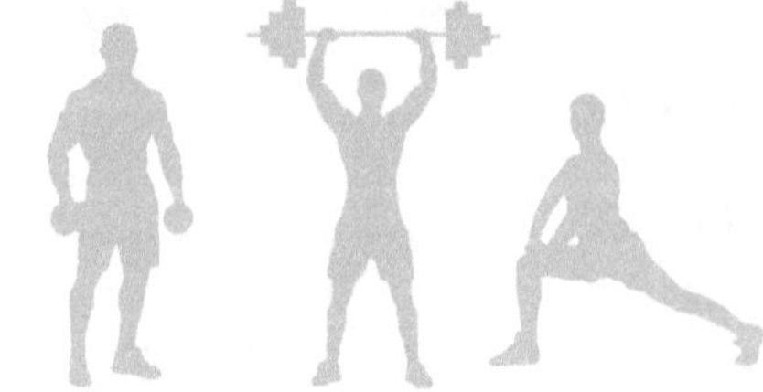

Name: ....

Date: ....

Time: ....

Warm-Up

ACTIVITY	TIME	REPS

 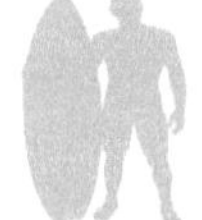 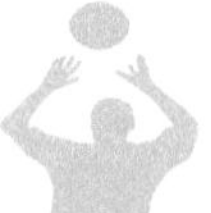 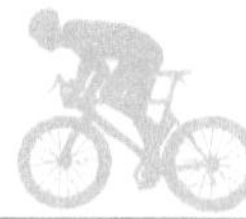

Cardio

ACTIVITY	DISTANCE	TIME	TARGET HEART RATE

Strength Training

EXERCISE	SET ONE WEIGHT/REPS	SET TWO WEIGHT/REPS	SET THREE WEIGHT/REPS

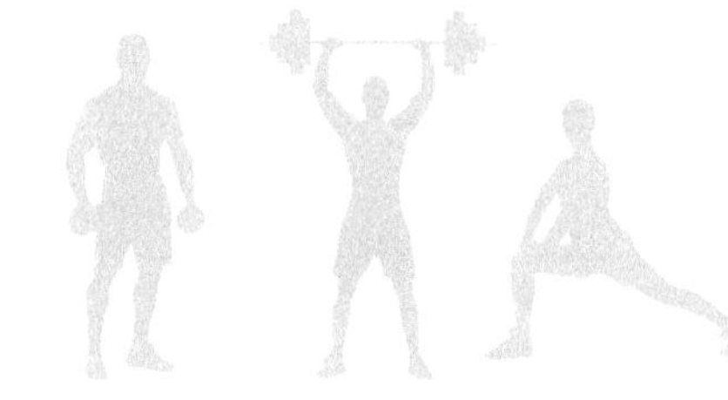

Name: ....

Date: ....

Time: ....

Warm-Up

ACTIVITY	TIME	REPS

Cardio

ACTIVITY	DISTANCE	TIME	TARGET HEART RATE

Strength Training

EXERCISE	SET ONE WEIGHT/REPS	SET TWO WEIGHT/REPS	SET THREE WEIGHT/REPS

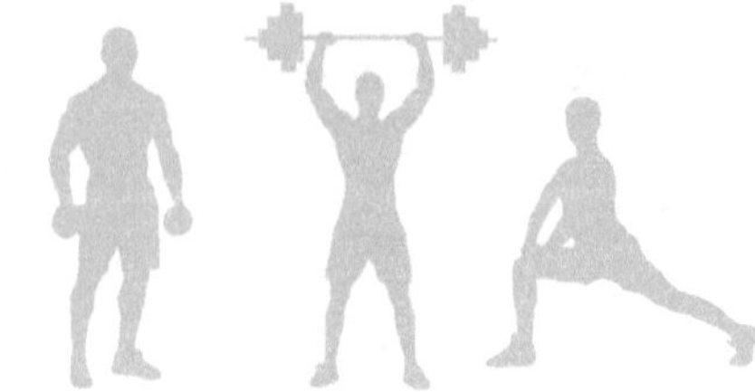

Name: ....

Date: ....

Time: ....

Warm-Up

ACTIVITY	TIME	REPS

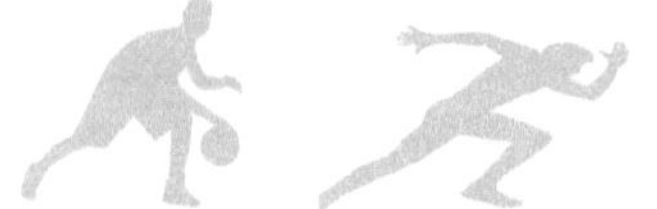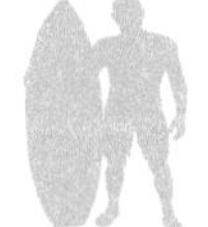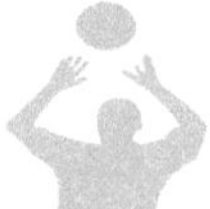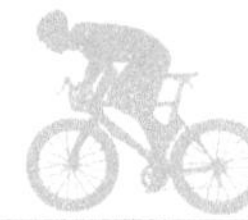

Cardio

ACTIVITY	DISTANCE	TIME	TARGET HEART RATE

Strength Training

EXERCISE	SET ONE WEIGHT/REPS	SET TWO WEIGHT/REPS	SET THREE WEIGHT/REPS

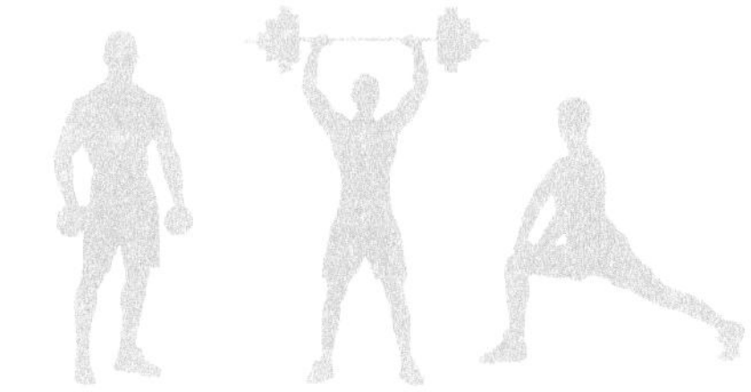

Name: ....

Date: ....

Time: ....

Warm-Up

ACTIVITY	TIME	REPS

Cardio

ACTIVITY	DISTANCE	TIME	TARGET HEART RATE

Strength Training

EXERCISE	SET ONE WEIGHT/REPS	SET TWO WEIGHT/REPS	SET THREE WEIGHT/REPS

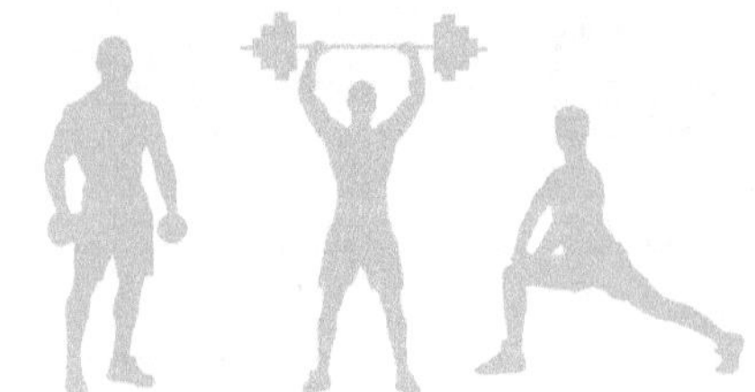

Name: ....

Date: ....

Time: ....

Warm-Up

ACTIVITY	TIME	REPS

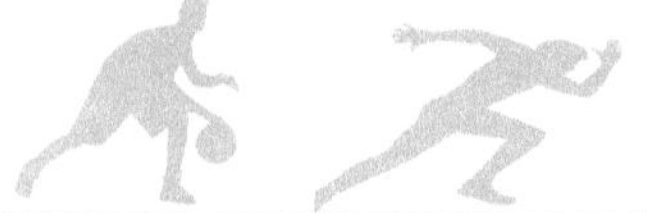 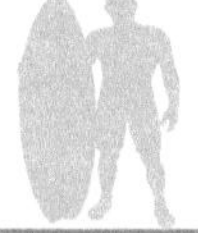 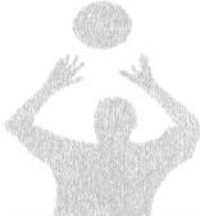 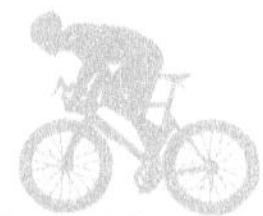

Cardio

ACTIVITY	DISTANCE	TIME	TARGET HEART RATE

Strength Training

EXERCISE	SET ONE WEIGHT/REPS	SET TWO WEIGHT/REPS	SET THREE WEIGHT/REPS

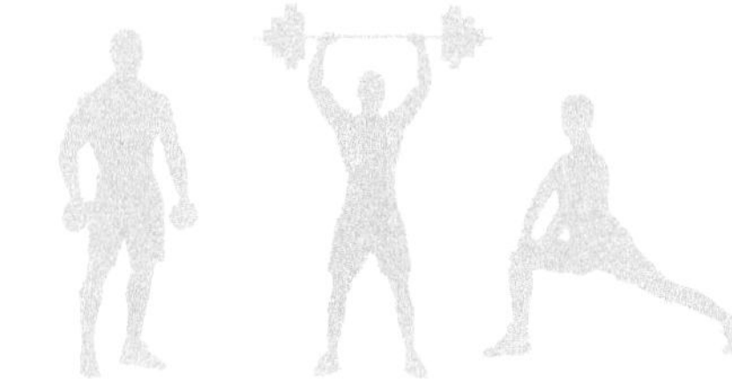

Name: ……………………….

Date: ……………………….

Time: ……………………….

Warm-Up

ACTIVITY	TIME	REPS

Cardio

ACTIVITY	DISTANCE	TIME	TARGET HEART RATE

Strength Training

EXERCISE	SET ONE WEIGHT/REPS	SET TWO WEIGHT/REPS	SET THREE WEIGHT/REPS

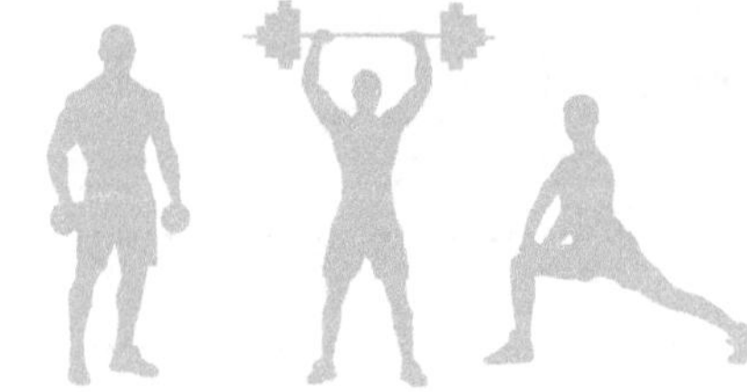

Name: ....

Date: ....

Time: ....

Warm-Up

ACTIVITY	TIME	REPS

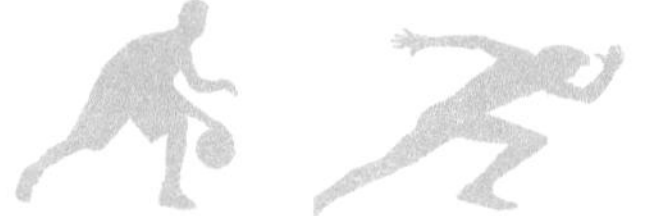 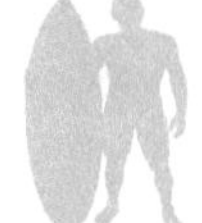 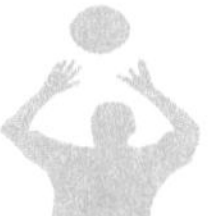 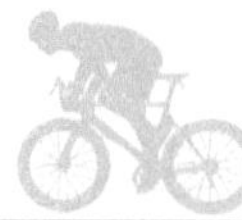

Cardio

ACTIVITY	DISTANCE	TIME	TARGET HEART RATE

Strength Training

EXERCISE	SET ONE WEIGHT/REPS	SET TWO WEIGHT/REPS	SET THREE WEIGHT/REPS

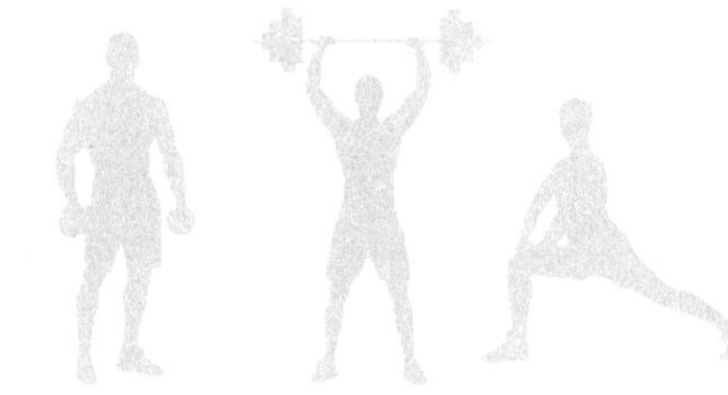

Name: ....

Date: ....

Time: ....

Warm-Up

ACTIVITY	TIME	REPS

Cardio

ACTIVITY	DISTANCE	TIME	TARGET HEART RATE

Strength Training

EXERCISE	SET ONE WEIGHT/REPS	SET TWO WEIGHT/REPS	SET THREE WEIGHT/REPS

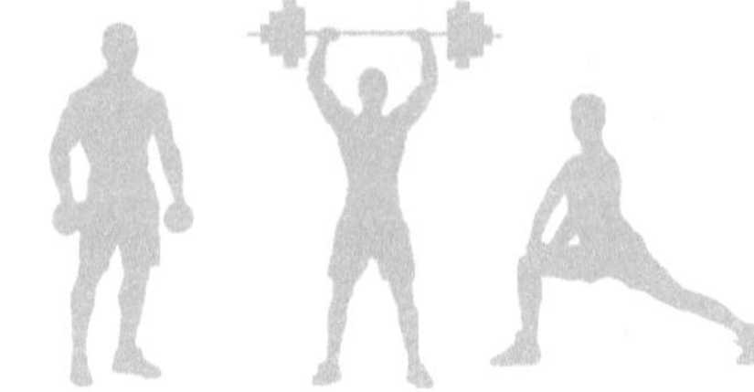

Name: ....

Date: ....

Time: ....

Warm-Up

ACTIVITY	TIME	REPS

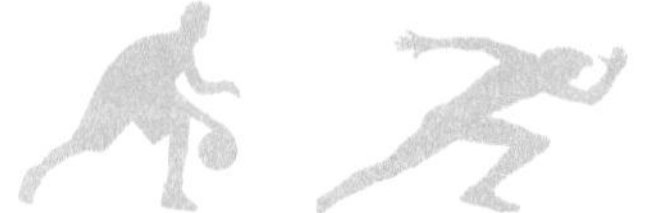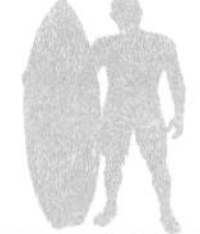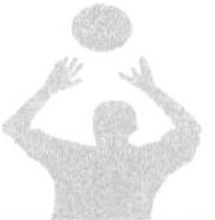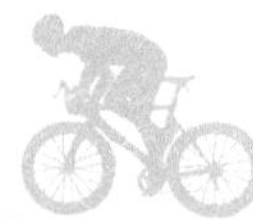

Cardio

ACTIVITY	DISTANCE	TIME	TARGET HEART RATE

Strength Training

EXERCISE	SET ONE WEIGHT/REPS	SET TWO WEIGHT/REPS	SET THREE WEIGHT/REPS

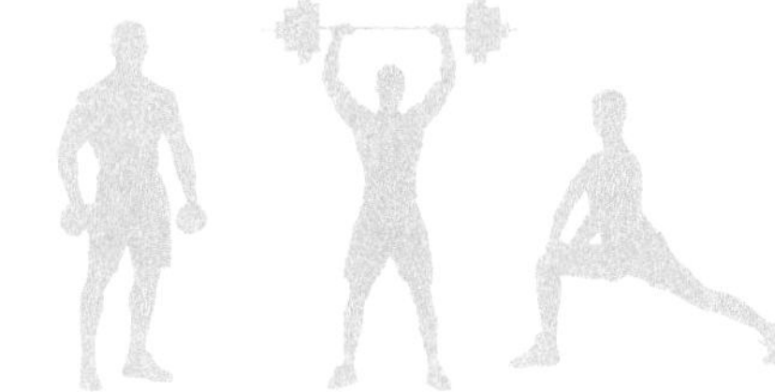

Name: ....

Date: ....

Time: ....

Warm-Up

ACTIVITY	TIME	REPS

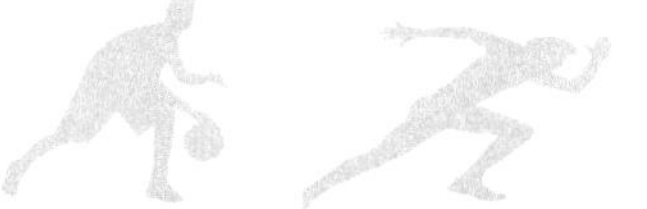 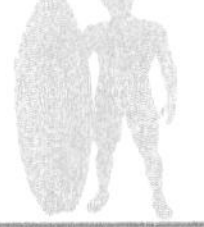 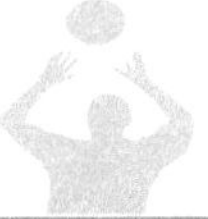 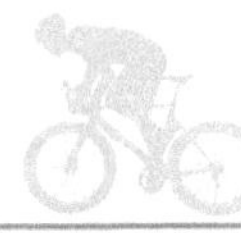

Cardio

ACTIVITY	DISTANCE	TIME	TARGET HEART RATE

Strength Training

EXERCISE	SET ONE WEIGHT/REPS	SET TWO WEIGHT/REPS	SET THREE WEIGHT/REPS

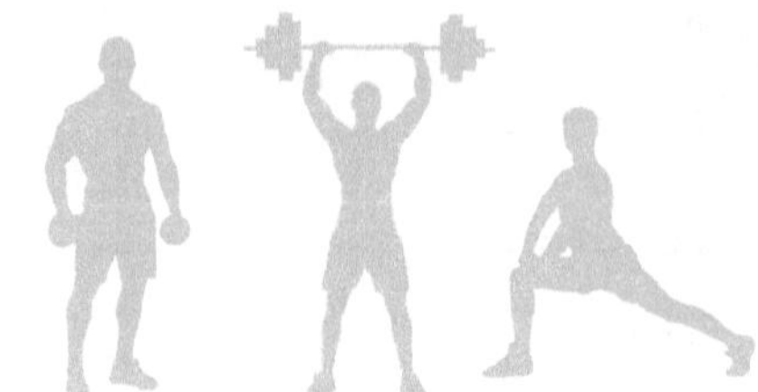

Name: ....

Date: ....

Time: ....

Warm-Up

ACTIVITY	TIME	REPS

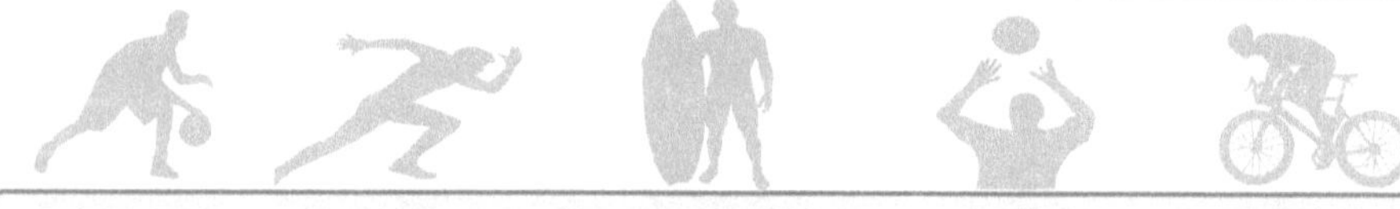

Cardio

ACTIVITY	DISTANCE	TIME	TARGET HEART RATE

Strength Training

EXERCISE	SET ONE WEIGHT/REPS	SET TWO WEIGHT/REPS	SET THREE WEIGHT/REPS

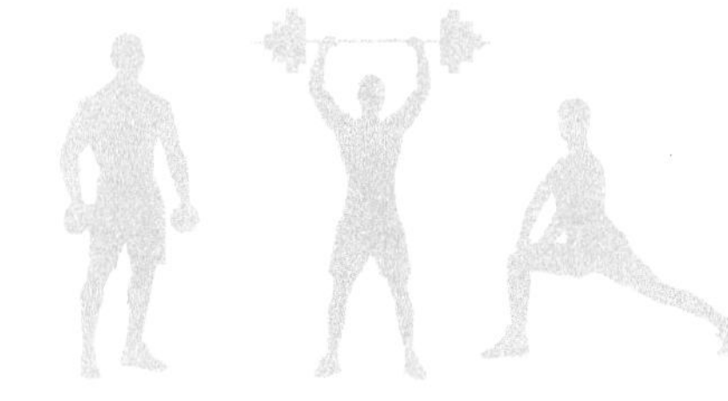

Name: ....

Date: ....

Time: ....

Warm-Up

ACTIVITY	TIME	REPS

Cardio

ACTIVITY	DISTANCE	TIME	TARGET HEART RATE

Strength Training

EXERCISE	SET ONE WEIGHT/REPS	SET TWO WEIGHT/REPS	SET THREE WEIGHT/REPS

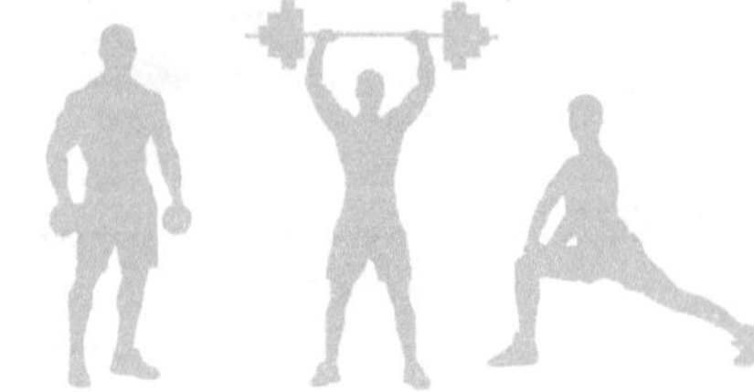

Name: ....

Date: ....

Time: ....

Warm-Up

ACTIVITY	TIME	REPS

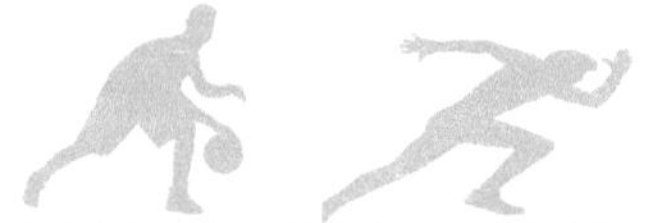 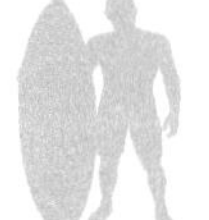 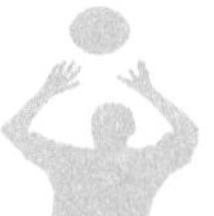 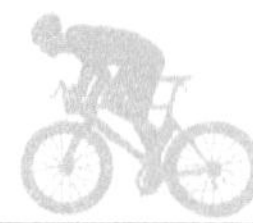

Cardio

ACTIVITY	DISTANCE	TIME	TARGET HEART RATE

Strength Training

EXERCISE	SET ONE WEIGHT/REPS	SET TWO WEIGHT/REPS	SET THREE WEIGHT/REPS

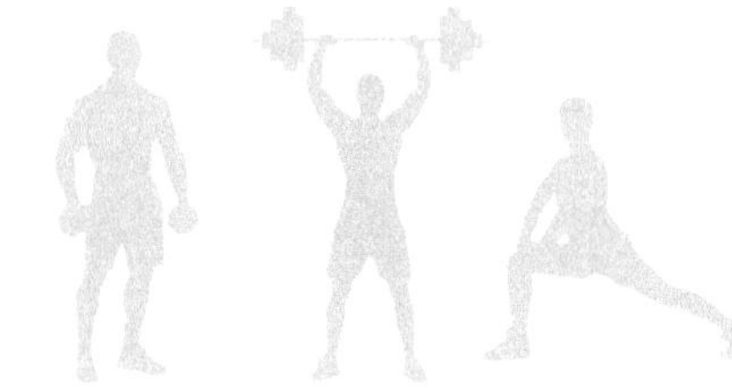

Name: ....

Date: ....

Time: ....

Warm-Up

ACTIVITY	TIME	REPS

Cardio

ACTIVITY	DISTANCE	TIME	TARGET HEART RATE

Strength Training

EXERCISE	SET ONE WEIGHT/REPS	SET TWO WEIGHT/REPS	SET THREE WEIGHT/REPS

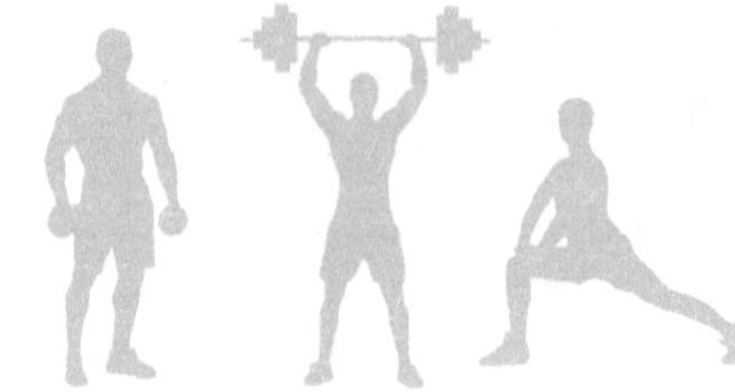

Name: ....

Date: ....

Time: ....

Warm-Up

ACTIVITY	TIME	REPS

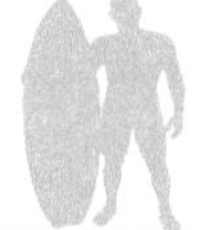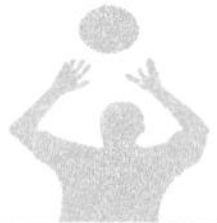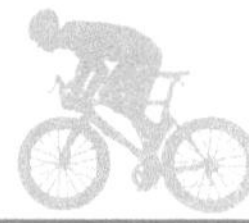

Cardio

ACTIVITY	DISTANCE	TIME	TARGET HEART RATE

Strength Training

EXERCISE	SET ONE WEIGHT/REPS	SET TWO WEIGHT/REPS	SET THREE WEIGHT/REPS

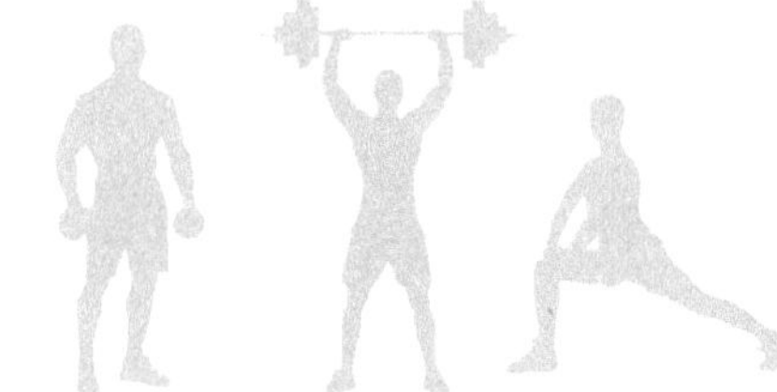

Name: ....

Date: ....

Time: ....

Warm-Up

ACTIVITY	TIME	REPS

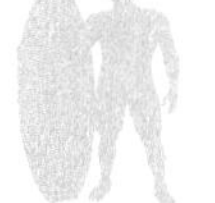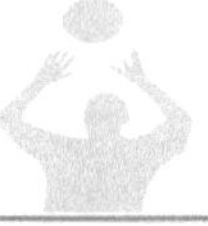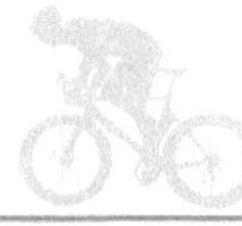

Cardio

ACTIVITY	DISTANCE	TIME	TARGET HEART RATE

Strength Training

EXERCISE	SET ONE WEIGHT/REPS	SET TWO WEIGHT/REPS	SET THREE WEIGHT/REPS

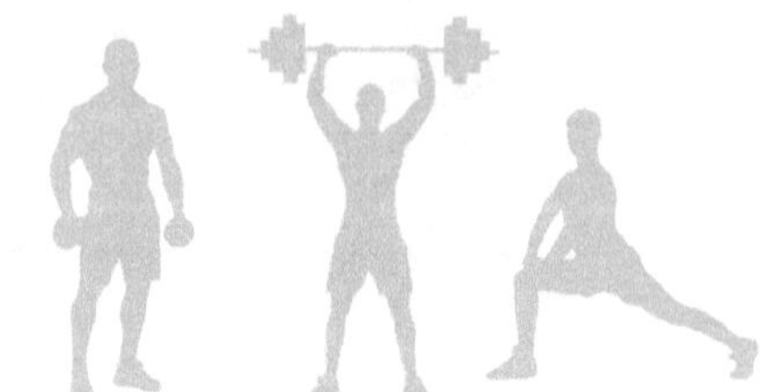

Name: ....

Date: ....

Time: ....

Warm-Up

ACTIVITY	TIME	REPS

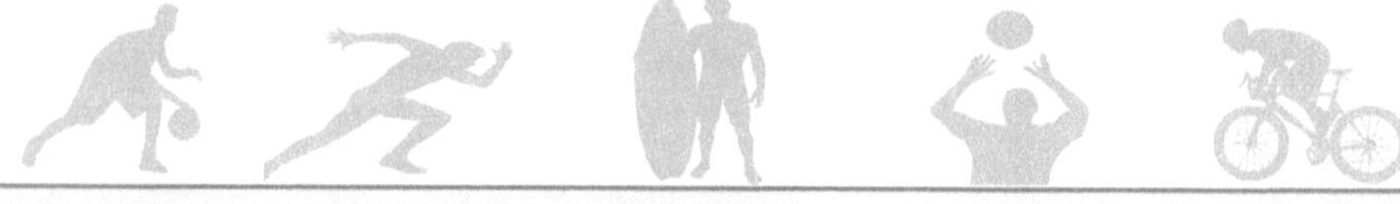

Cardio

ACTIVITY	DISTANCE	TIME	TARGET HEART RATE

Strength Training

EXERCISE	SET ONE WEIGHT/REPS	SET TWO WEIGHT/REPS	SET THREE WEIGHT/REPS

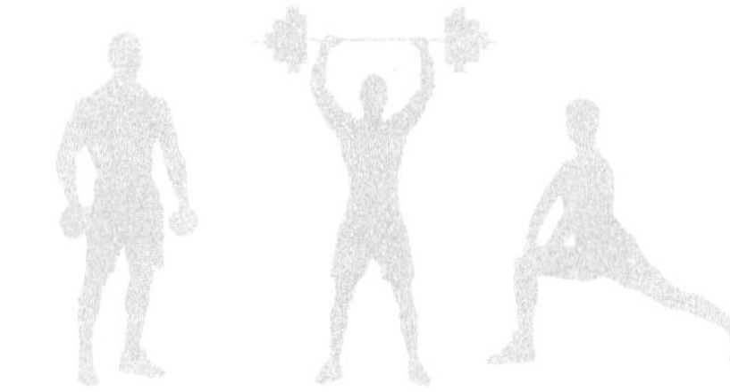

Name: ....

Date: ....

Time: ....

Warm-Up

ACTIVITY	TIME	REPS

Cardio

ACTIVITY	DISTANCE	TIME	TARGET HEART RATE

Strength Training

EXERCISE	SET ONE WEIGHT/REPS	SET TWO WEIGHT/REPS	SET THREE WEIGHT/REPS

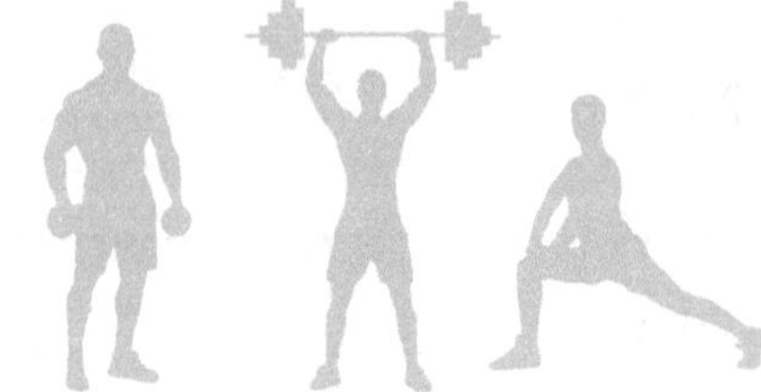

Name: ……………………………

Date: ……………………………

Time: ……………………………

Warm-Up

ACTIVITY	TIME	REPS

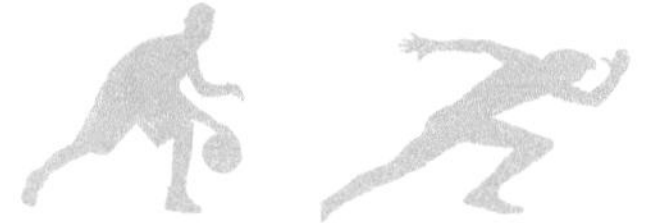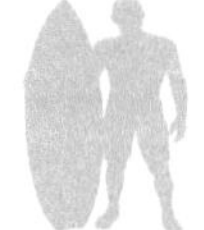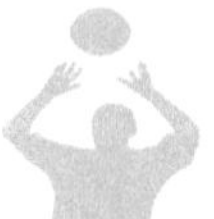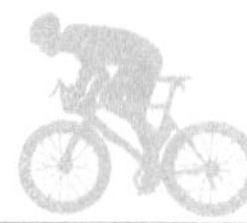

Cardio

ACTIVITY	DISTANCE	TIME	TARGET HEART RATE

Strength Training

EXERCISE	SET ONE WEIGHT/REPS	SET TWO WEIGHT/REPS	SET THREE WEIGHT/REPS

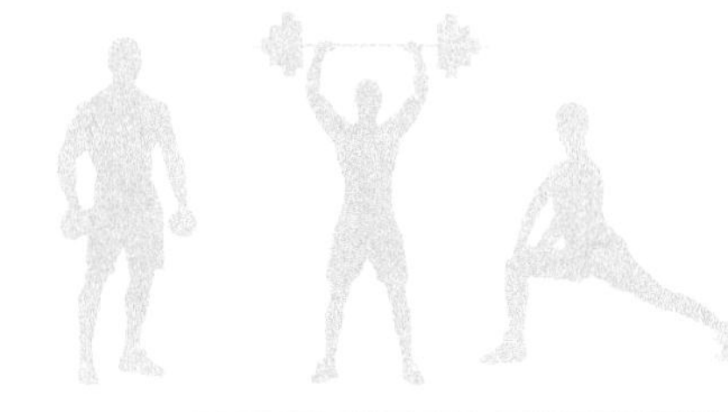

Warm-Up

ACTIVITY	TIME	REPS

Cardio

ACTIVITY	DISTANCE	TIME	TARGET HEART RATE

Strength Training

EXERCISE	SET ONE WEIGHT/REPS	SET TWO WEIGHT/REPS	SET THREE WEIGHT/REPS

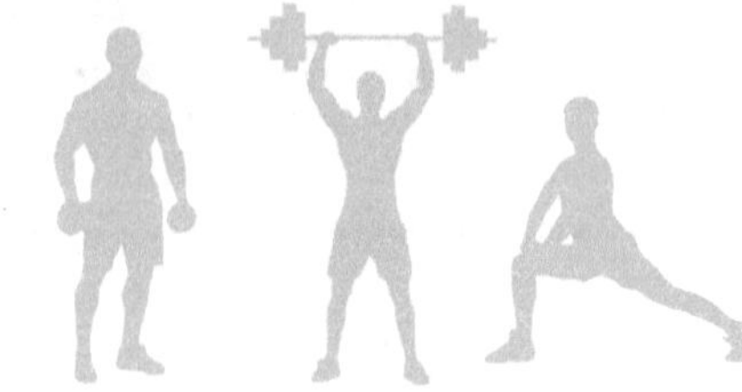

Name: ....

Date: ....

Time: ....

Warm-Up

ACTIVITY	TIME	REPS

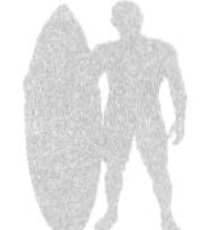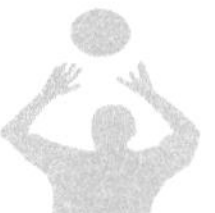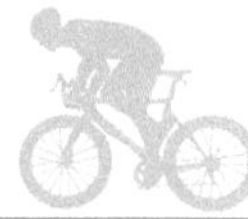

Cardio

ACTIVITY	DISTANCE	TIME	TARGET HEART RATE

Strength Training

EXERCISE	SET ONE WEIGHT/REPS	SET TWO WEIGHT/REPS	SET THREE WEIGHT/REPS

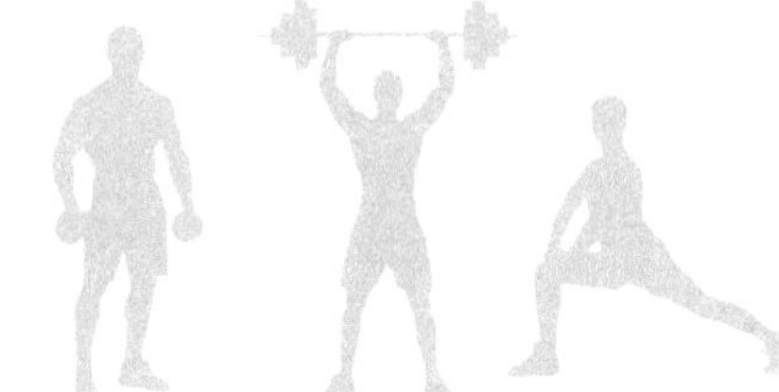

Name: ....

Date: ....

Time: ....

Warm-Up

ACTIVITY	TIME	REPS

 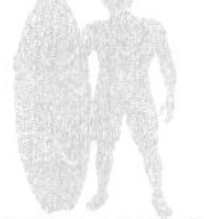 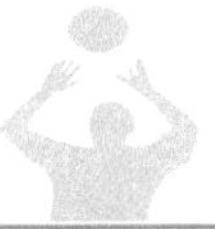 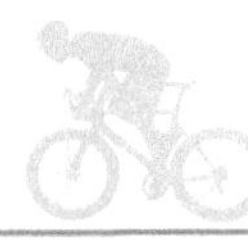

Cardio

ACTIVITY	DISTANCE	TIME	TARGET HEART RATE

Strength Training

EXERCISE	SET ONE WEIGHT/REPS	SET TWO WEIGHT/REPS	SET THREE WEIGHT/REPS

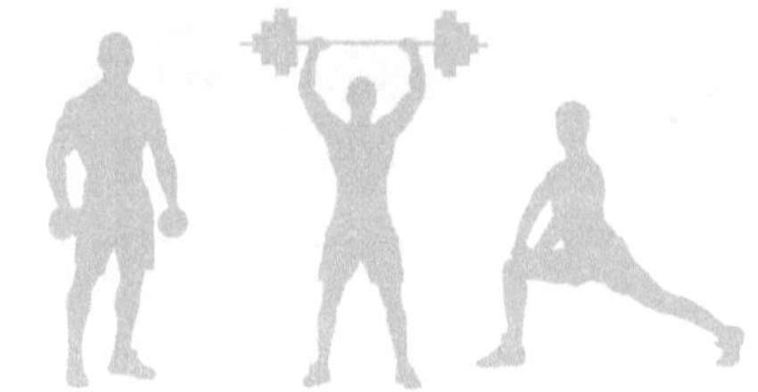

Name: ....

Date: ....

Time: ....

Warm-Up

ACTIVITY	TIME	REPS

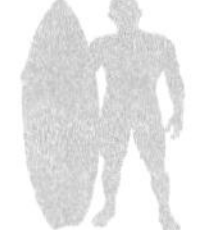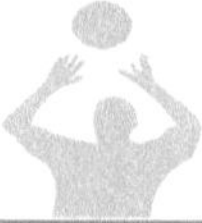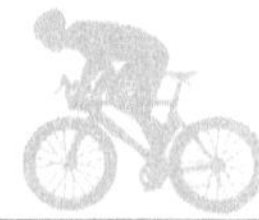

Cardio

ACTIVITY	DISTANCE	TIME	TARGET HEART RATE

Strength Training

EXERCISE	SET ONE WEIGHT/REPS	SET TWO WEIGHT/REPS	SET THREE WEIGHT/REPS

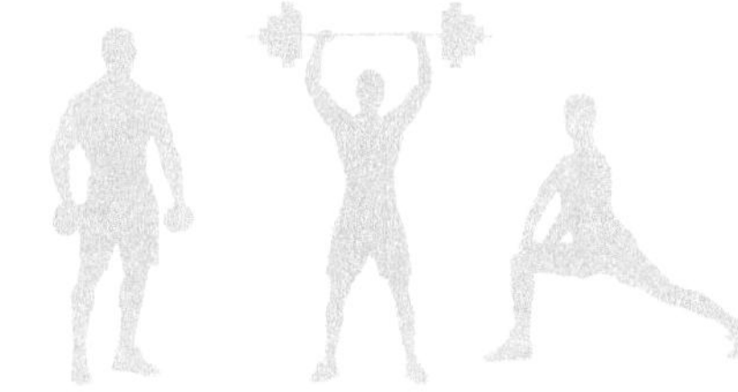

Name: ....

Date: ....

Time: ....

Warm-Up

ACTIVITY	TIME	REPS

Cardio

ACTIVITY	DISTANCE	TIME	TARGET HEART RATE

Strength Training

EXERCISE	SET ONE WEIGHT/REPS	SET TWO WEIGHT/REPS	SET THREE WEIGHT/REPS

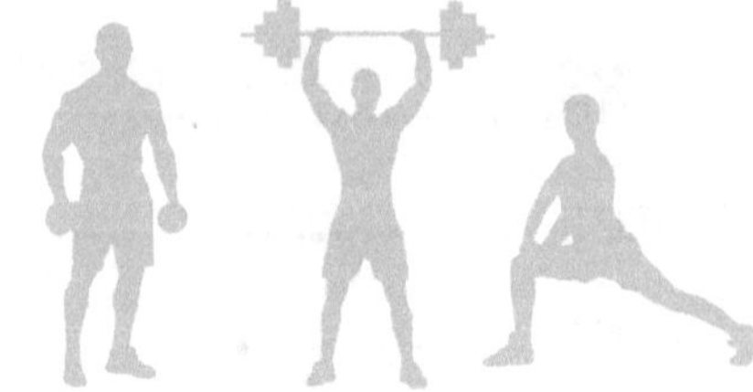

Name: ....

Date: ....

Time: ....

Warm-Up

ACTIVITY	TIME	REPS

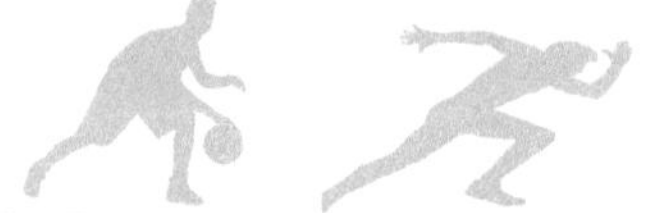 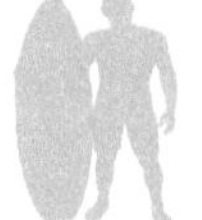 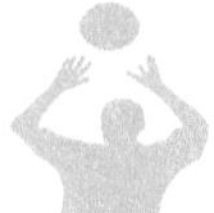 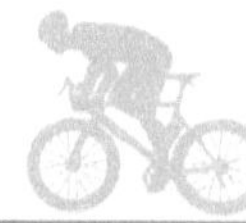

Cardio

ACTIVITY	DISTANCE	TIME	TARGET HEART RATE

Strength Training

EXERCISE	SET ONE WEIGHT/REPS	SET TWO WEIGHT/REPS	SET THREE WEIGHT/REPS

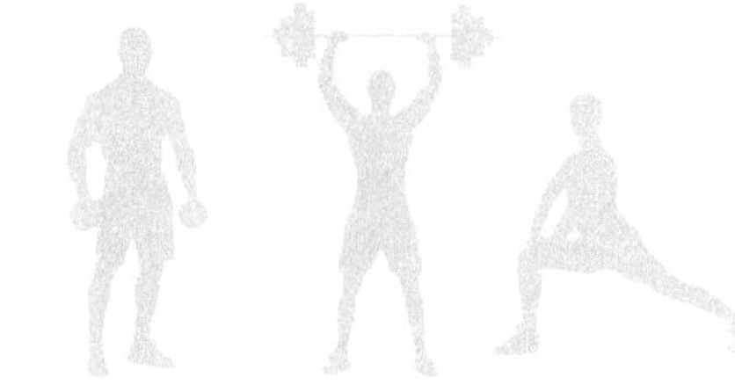

Name: …………………………….

Date: …………………………….

Time: …………………………….

Warm-Up

ACTIVITY	TIME	REPS

Cardio

ACTIVITY	DISTANCE	TIME	TARGET HEART RATE

Strength Training

EXERCISE	SET ONE WEIGHT/REPS	SET TWO WEIGHT/REPS	SET THREE WEIGHT/REPS

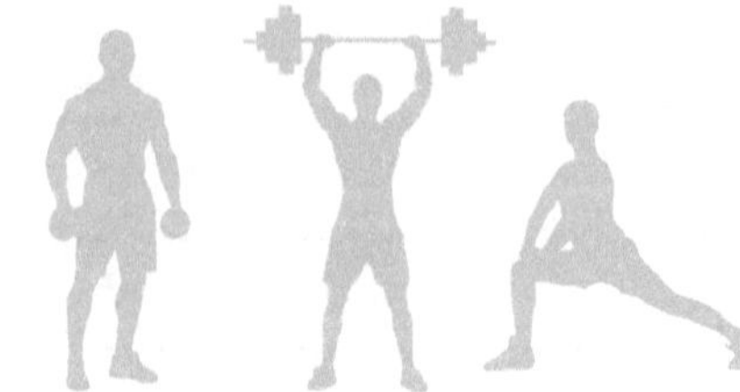

Name: ....

Date: ....

Time: ....

Warm-Up

ACTIVITY	TIME	REPS

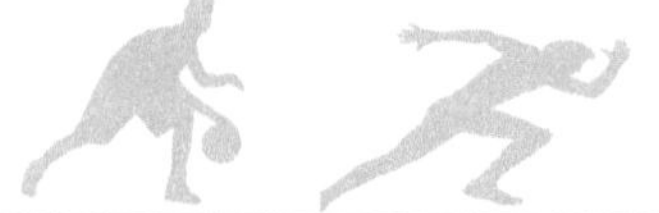 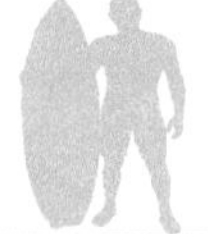 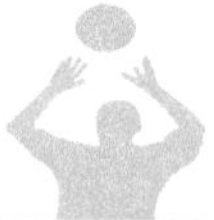 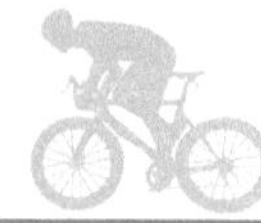

Cardio

ACTIVITY	DISTANCE	TIME	TARGET HEART RATE

Strength Training

EXERCISE	SET ONE WEIGHT/REPS	SET TWO WEIGHT/REPS	SET THREE WEIGHT/REPS

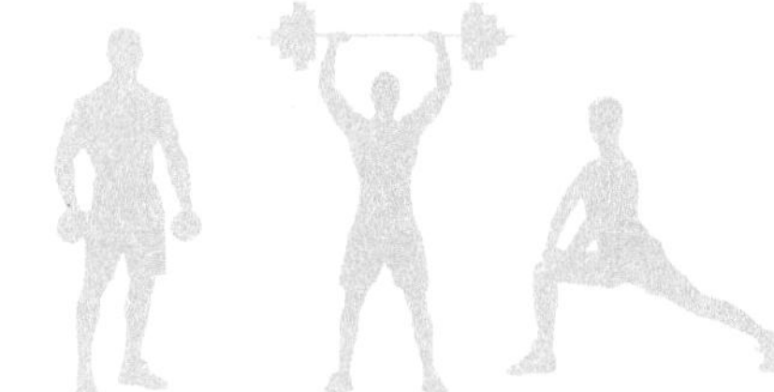

Name: ....

Date: ....

Time: ....

Warm-Up

ACTIVITY	TIME	REPS

Cardio

ACTIVITY	DISTANCE	TIME	TARGET HEART RATE

Strength Training

EXERCISE 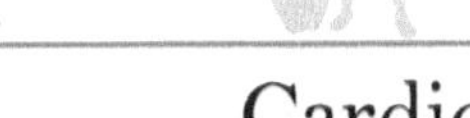	SET ONE WEIGHT/REPS	SET TWO WEIGHT/REPS	SET THREE WEIGHT/REPS

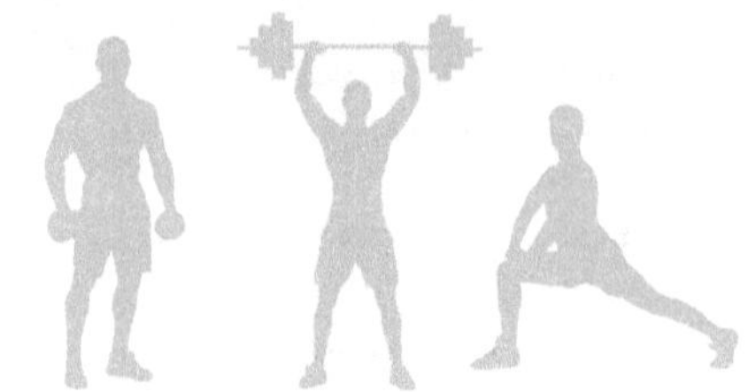

Name: ....

Date: ....

Time: ....

Warm-Up

ACTIVITY	TIME	REPS

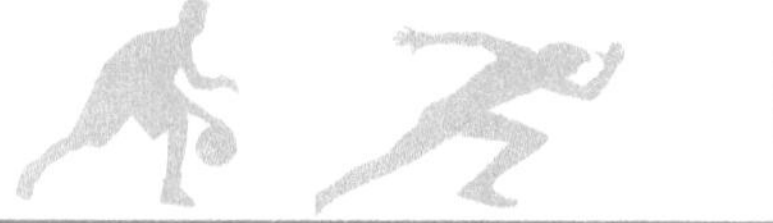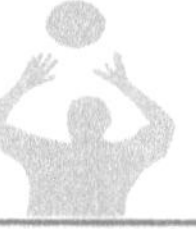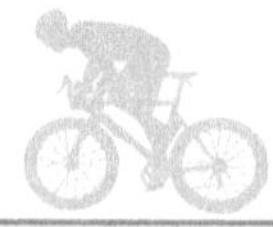

Cardio

ACTIVITY	DISTANCE	TIME	TARGET HEART RATE

Strength Training

EXERCISE	SET ONE WEIGHT/REPS	SET TWO WEIGHT/REPS	SET THREE WEIGHT/REPS

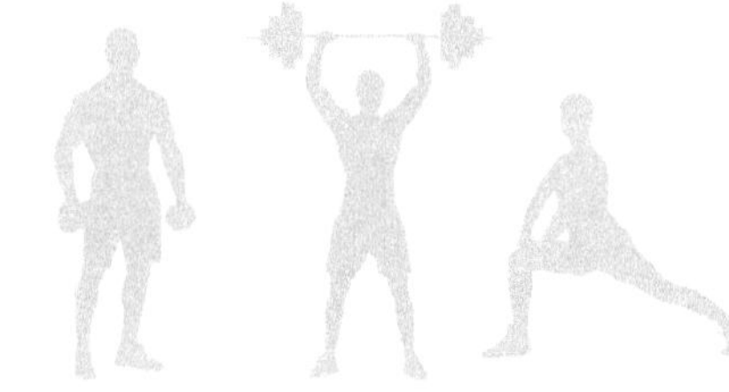

Name: ………………………………

Date: ………………………………

Time: ………………………………

Warm-Up

ACTIVITY	TIME	REPS

Cardio

ACTIVITY	DISTANCE	TIME	TARGET HEART RATE

Strength Training

EXERCISE	SET ONE WEIGHT/REPS	SET TWO WEIGHT/REPS	SET THREE WEIGHT/REPS

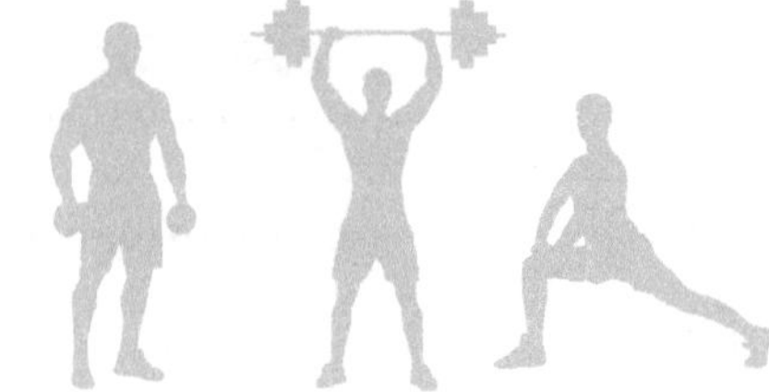

Name: ....

Date: ....

Time: ....

Warm-Up

ACTIVITY	TIME	REPS

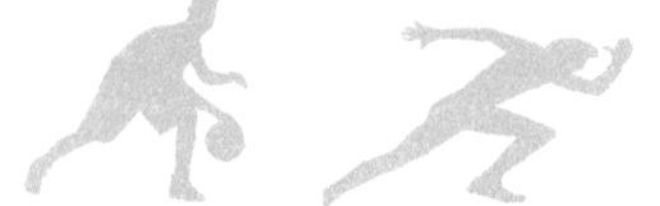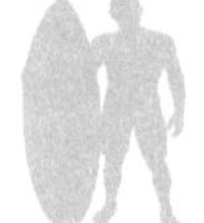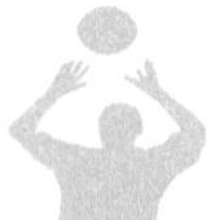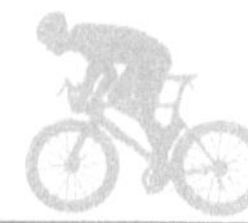

Cardio

ACTIVITY	DISTANCE	TIME	TARGET HEART RATE

Strength Training

EXERCISE	SET ONE WEIGHT/REPS	SET TWO WEIGHT/REPS	SET THREE WEIGHT/REPS

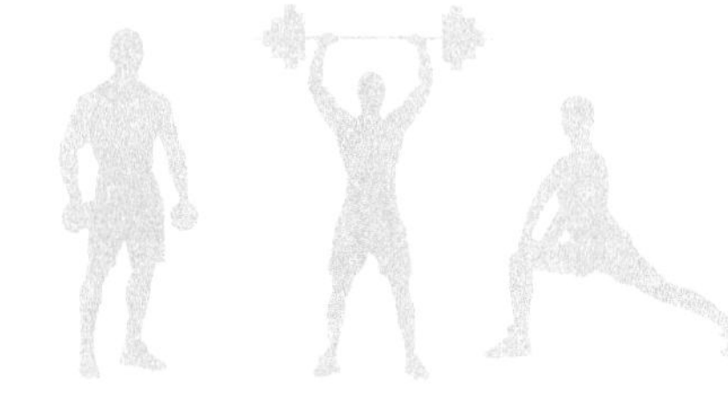

Name: ....

Date: ....

Time: ....

Warm-Up

ACTIVITY	TIME	REPS

Cardio

ACTIVITY	DISTANCE	TIME	TARGET HEART RATE

Strength Training

EXERCISE	SET ONE WEIGHT/REPS	SET TWO WEIGHT/REPS	SET THREE WEIGHT/REPS

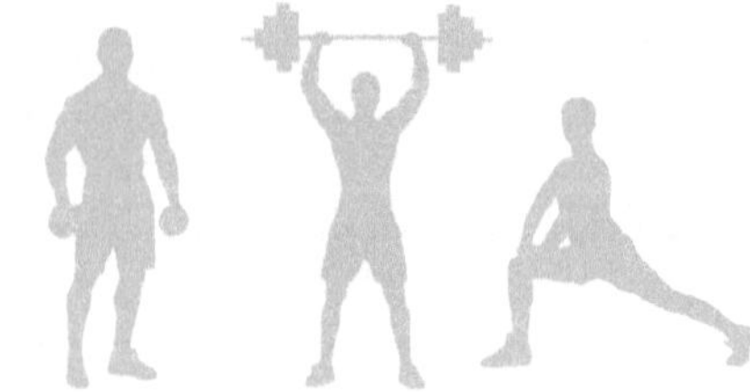

Name: ....

Date: ....

Time: ....

Warm-Up

ACTIVITY	TIME	REPS

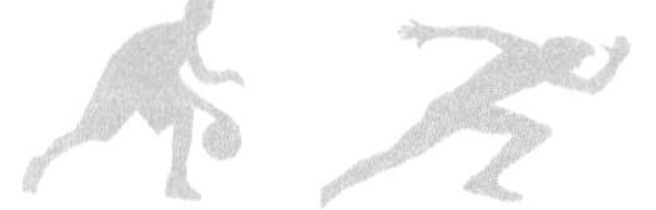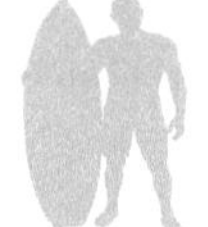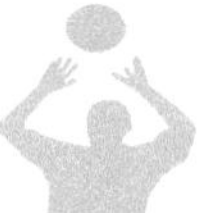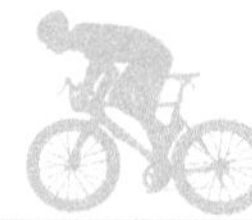

Cardio

ACTIVITY	DISTANCE	TIME	TARGET HEART RATE

Strength Training

EXERCISE	SET ONE WEIGHT/REPS	SET TWO WEIGHT/REPS	SET THREE WEIGHT/REPS

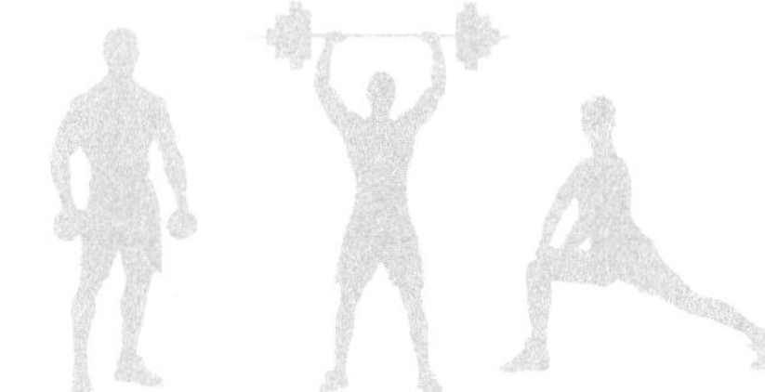

Name: ....

Date: ....

Time: ....

Warm-Up

ACTIVITY	TIME	REPS

 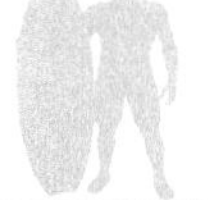 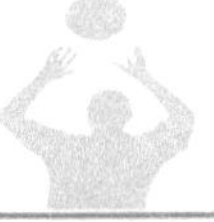 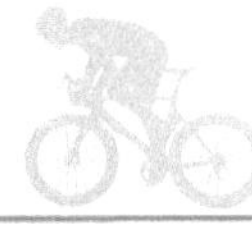

Cardio

ACTIVITY	DISTANCE	TIME	TARGET HEART RATE

Strength Training

EXERCISE	SET ONE WEIGHT/REPS	SET TWO WEIGHT/REPS	SET THREE WEIGHT/REPS

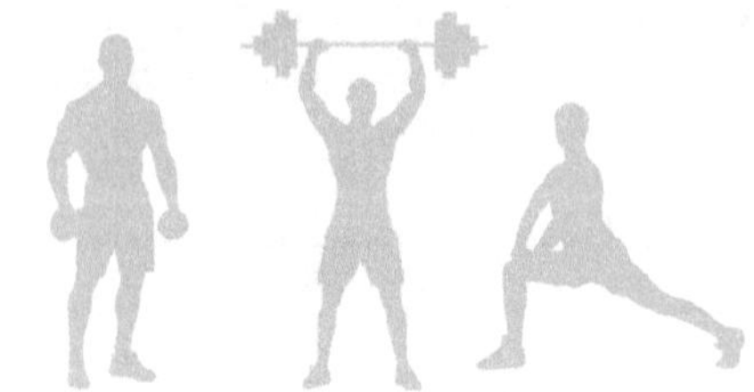

Name: ....

Date: ....

Time: ....

Warm-Up

ACTIVITY	TIME	REPS

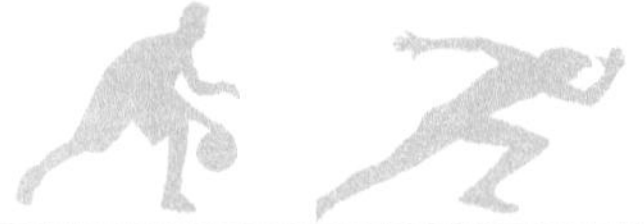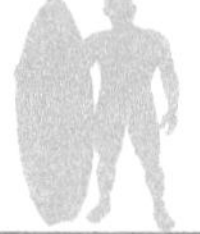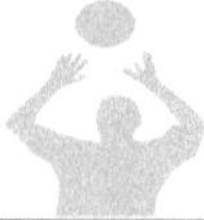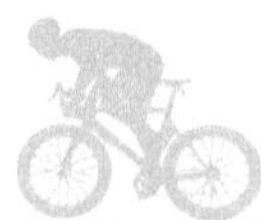

Cardio

ACTIVITY	DISTANCE	TIME	TARGET HEART RATE

Strength Training

EXERCISE	SET ONE WEIGHT/REPS	SET TWO WEIGHT/REPS	SET THREE WEIGHT/REPS

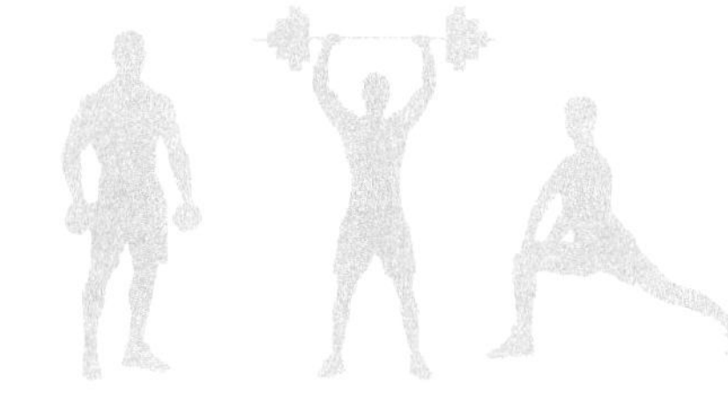

Name: ....

Date: ....

Time: ....

Warm-Up

ACTIVITY	TIME	REPS

Cardio

ACTIVITY	DISTANCE	TIME	TARGET HEART RATE

Strength Training

EXERCISE	SET ONE WEIGHT/REPS	SET TWO WEIGHT/REPS	SET THREE WEIGHT/REPS

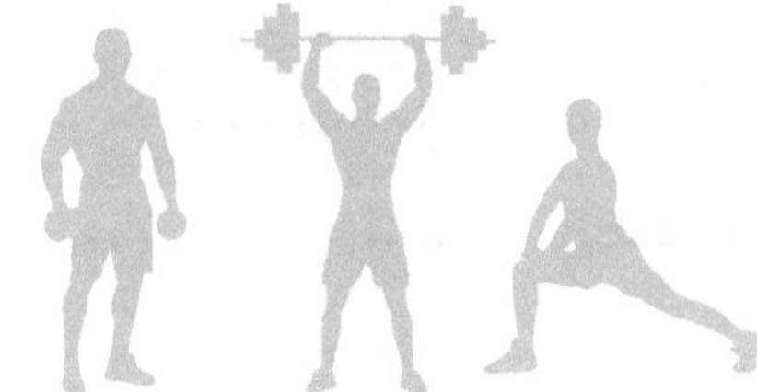

Name: ....

Date: ....

Time: ....

Warm-Up

ACTIVITY	TIME	REPS

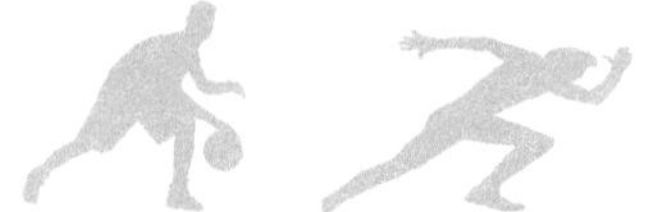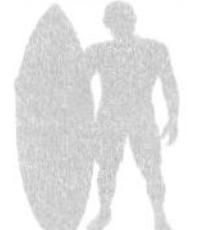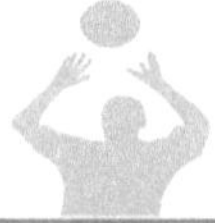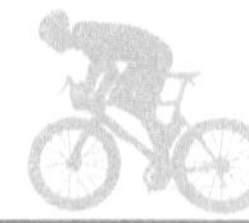

Cardio

ACTIVITY	DISTANCE	TIME	TARGET HEART RATE

Strength Training

EXERCISE	SET ONE WEIGHT/REPS	SET TWO WEIGHT/REPS	SET THREE WEIGHT/REPS

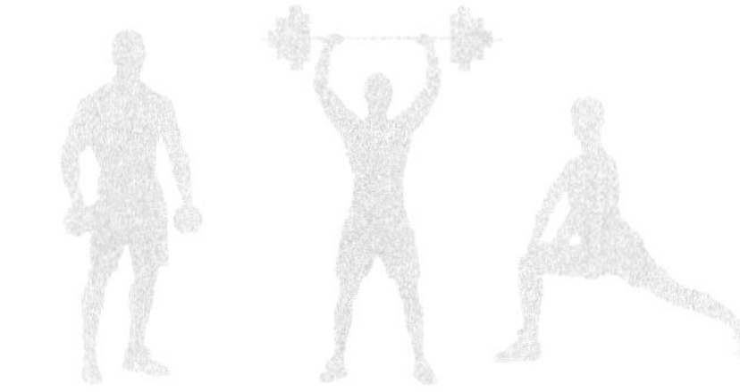

Warm-Up

ACTIVITY	TIME	REPS

Cardio

ACTIVITY	DISTANCE	TIME	TARGET HEART RATE

Strength Training

EXERCISE	SET ONE WEIGHT/REPS	SET TWO WEIGHT/REPS	SET THREE WEIGHT/REPS

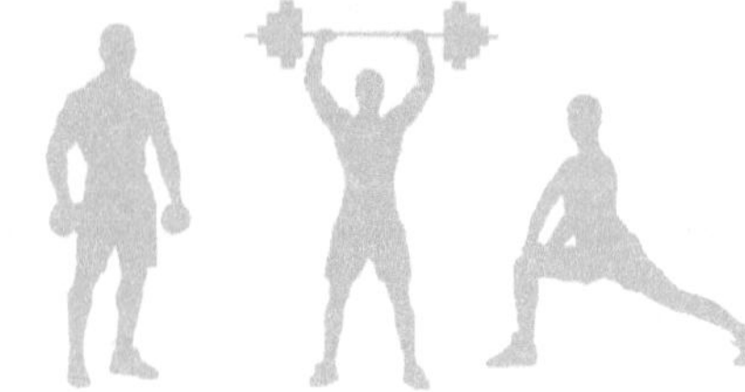

Warm-Up

ACTIVITY	TIME	REPS

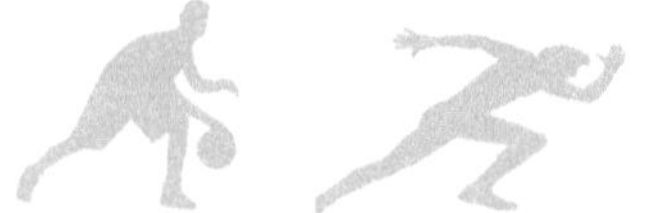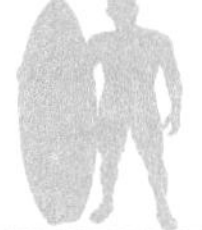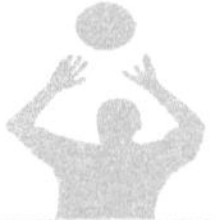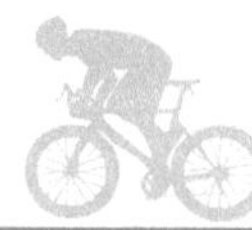

Cardio

ACTIVITY	DISTANCE	TIME	TARGET HEART RATE

Strength Training

EXERCISE	SET ONE WEIGHT/REPS	SET TWO WEIGHT/REPS	SET THREE WEIGHT/REPS

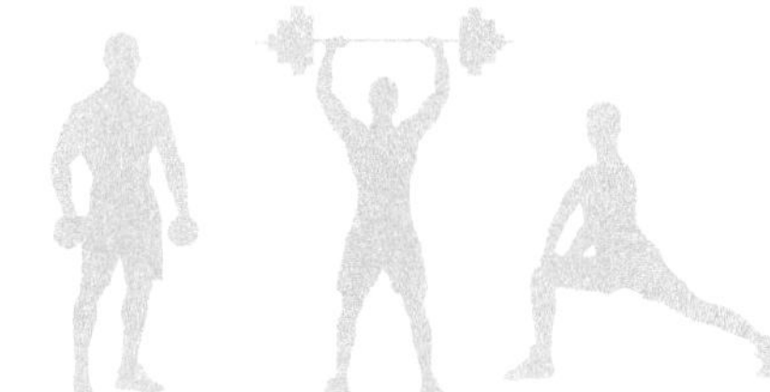

Warm-Up

ACTIVITY	TIME	REPS

Cardio

ACTIVITY	DISTANCE	TIME	TARGET HEART RATE

Strength Training

EXERCISE	SET ONE WEIGHT/REPS	SET TWO WEIGHT/REPS	SET THREE WEIGHT/REPS

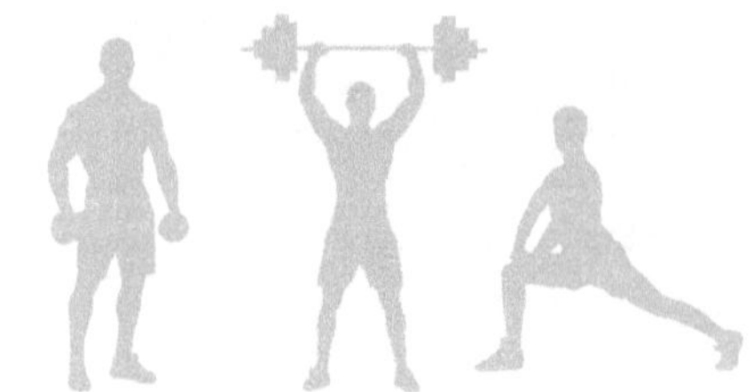

Name: ....

Date: ....

Time: ....

Warm-Up

ACTIVITY	TIME	REPS

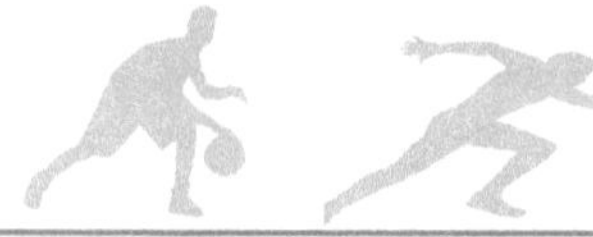 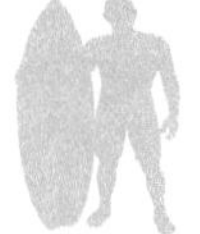 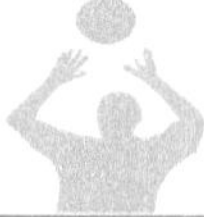 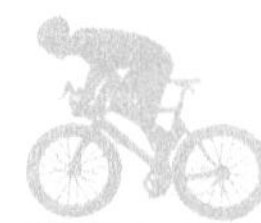

Cardio

ACTIVITY	DISTANCE	TIME	TARGET HEART RATE

Strength Training

EXERCISE	SET ONE WEIGHT/REPS	SET TWO WEIGHT/REPS	SET THREE WEIGHT/REPS

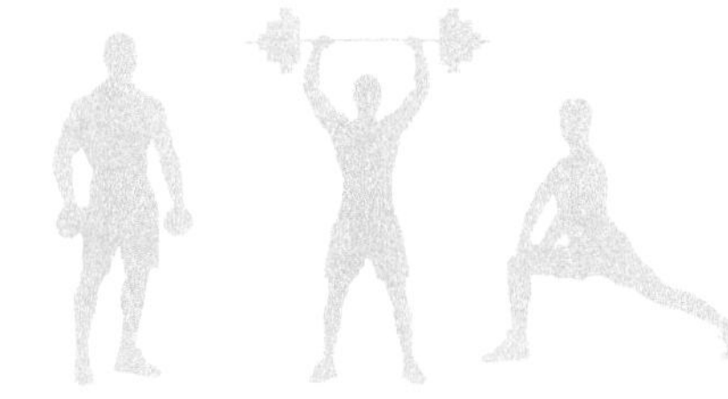

Name: ....

Date: ....

Time: ....

Warm-Up

ACTIVITY	TIME	REPS

Cardio

ACTIVITY	DISTANCE	TIME	TARGET HEART RATE

Strength Training

EXERCISE	SET ONE WEIGHT/REPS	SET TWO WEIGHT/REPS	SET THREE WEIGHT/REPS

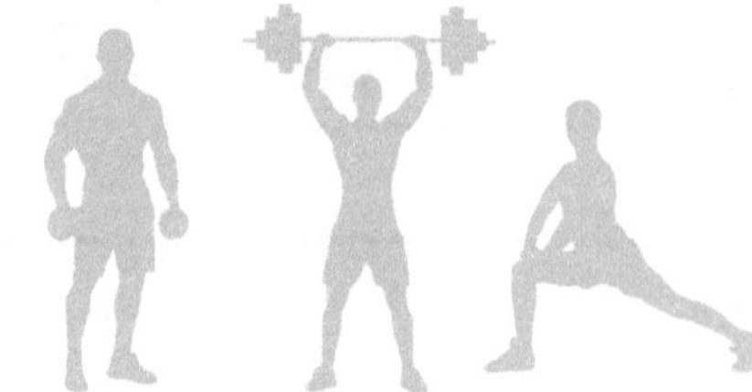

Name: ....

Date: ....

Time: ....

Warm-Up

ACTIVITY	TIME	REPS

 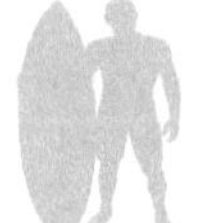 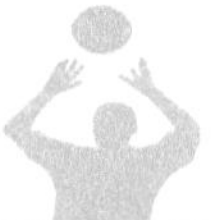 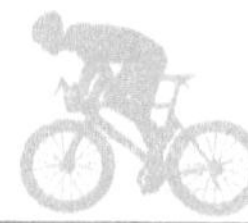

Cardio

ACTIVITY	DISTANCE	TIME	TARGET HEART RATE

Strength Training

EXERCISE	SET ONE WEIGHT/REPS	SET TWO WEIGHT/REPS	SET THREE WEIGHT/REPS

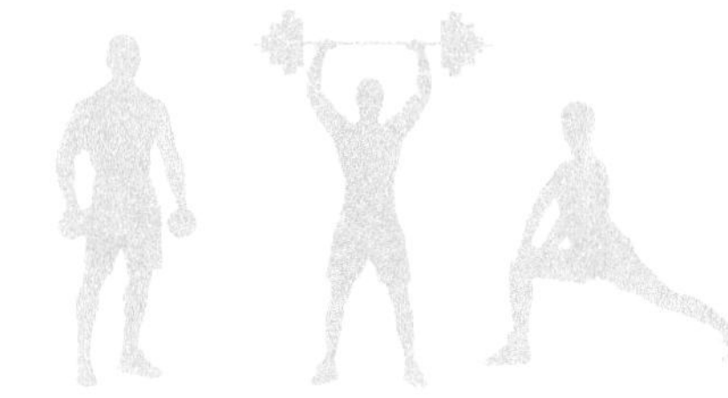

Name: ....

Date: ....

Time: ....

Warm-Up

ACTIVITY	TIME	REPS

Cardio

ACTIVITY	DISTANCE	TIME	TARGET HEART RATE

Strength Training

EXERCISE	SET ONE WEIGHT/REPS	SET TWO WEIGHT/REPS	SET THREE WEIGHT/REPS

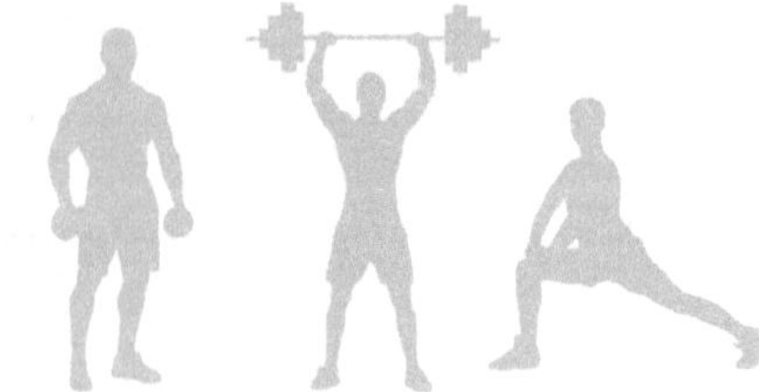

Name: ....

Date: ....

Time: ....

Warm-Up

ACTIVITY	TIME	REPS

 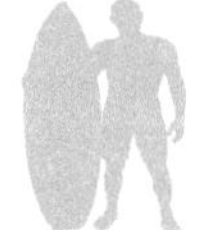 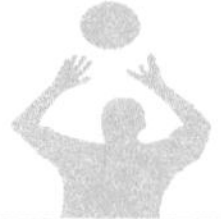 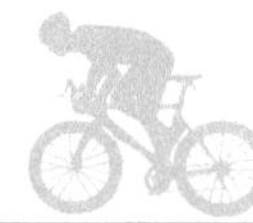

Cardio

ACTIVITY	DISTANCE	TIME	TARGET HEART RATE

Strength Training

EXERCISE	SET ONE WEIGHT/REPS	SET TWO WEIGHT/REPS	SET THREE WEIGHT/REPS

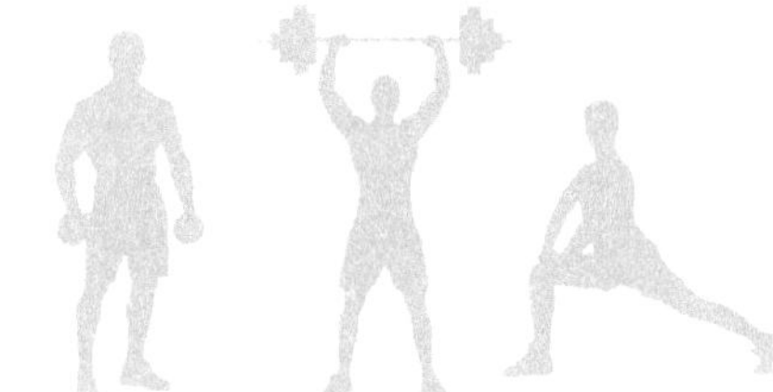

Name: ....

Date: ....

Time: ....

Warm-Up

ACTIVITY	TIME	REPS

Cardio

ACTIVITY	DISTANCE	TIME	TARGET HEART RATE

Strength Training

EXERCISE	SET ONE WEIGHT/REPS	SET TWO WEIGHT/REPS	SET THREE WEIGHT/REPS

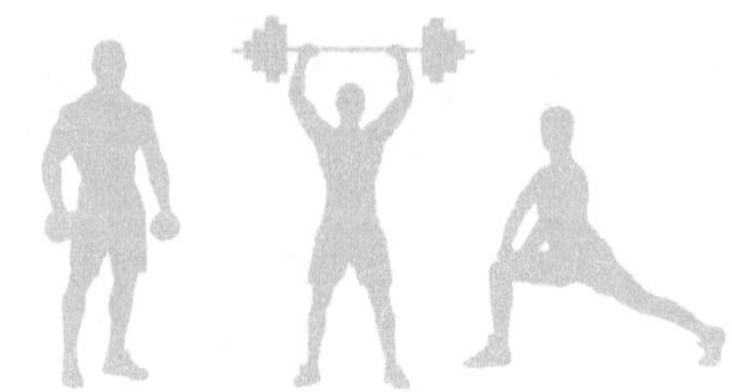

Name: ....

Date: ....

Time: ....

Warm-Up

ACTIVITY	TIME	REPS

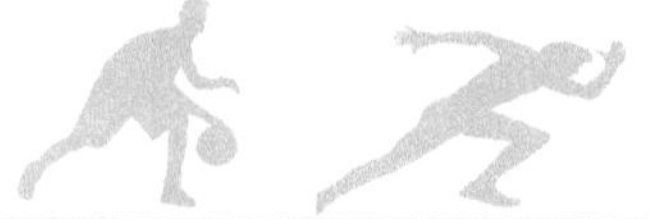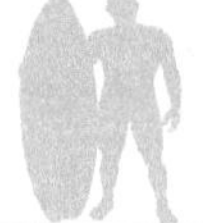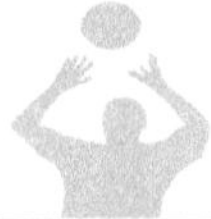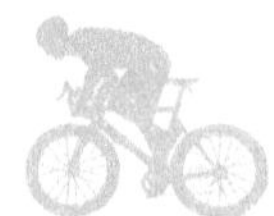

Cardio

ACTIVITY	DISTANCE	TIME	TARGET HEART RATE

Strength Training

EXERCISE	SET ONE WEIGHT/REPS	SET TWO WEIGHT/REPS	SET THREE WEIGHT/REPS

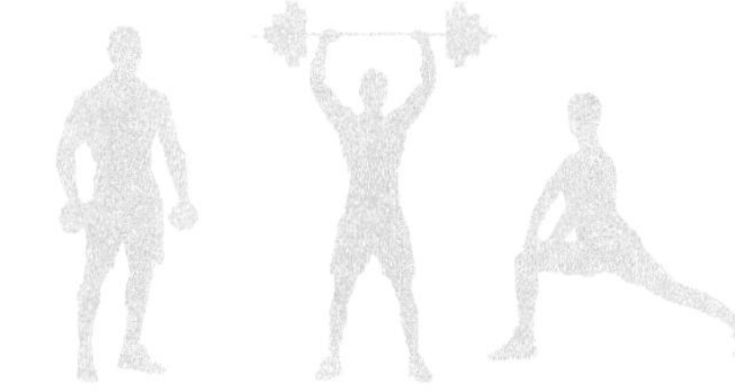

Name: ....

Date: ....

Time: ....

Warm-Up

ACTIVITY	TIME	REPS

Cardio

ACTIVITY	DISTANCE	TIME	TARGET HEART RATE

Strength Training

EXERCISE	SET ONE WEIGHT/REPS	SET TWO WEIGHT/REPS	SET THREE WEIGHT/REPS

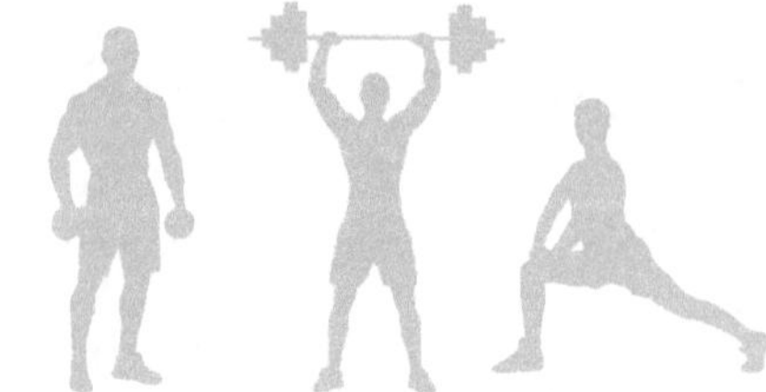

Name: ....

Date: ....

Time: ....

Warm-Up

ACTIVITY	TIME	REPS

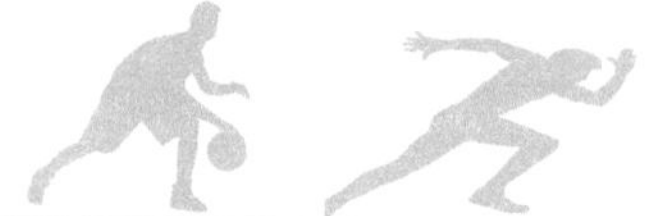 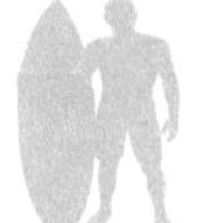 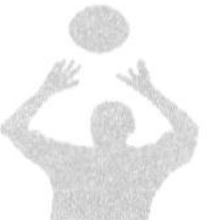 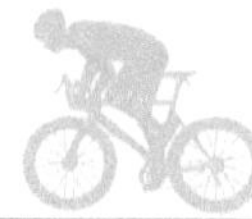

Cardio

ACTIVITY	DISTANCE	TIME	TARGET HEART RATE

Strength Training

EXERCISE	SET ONE WEIGHT/REPS	SET TWO WEIGHT/REPS	SET THREE WEIGHT/REPS

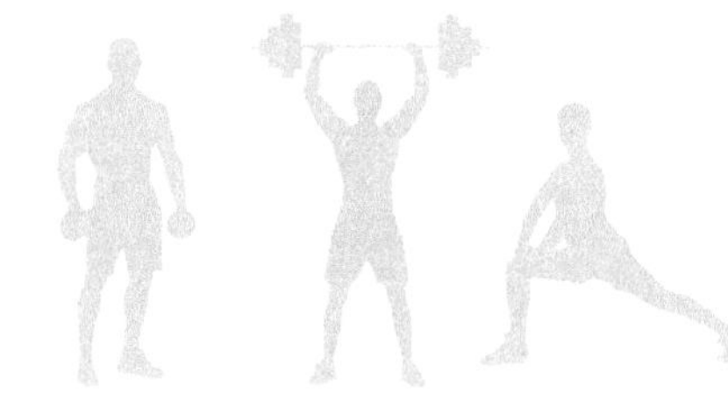

Warm-Up

ACTIVITY	TIME	REPS

Cardio

ACTIVITY	DISTANCE	TIME	TARGET HEART RATE

Strength Training

EXERCISE	SET ONE WEIGHT/REPS	SET TWO WEIGHT/REPS	SET THREE WEIGHT/REPS

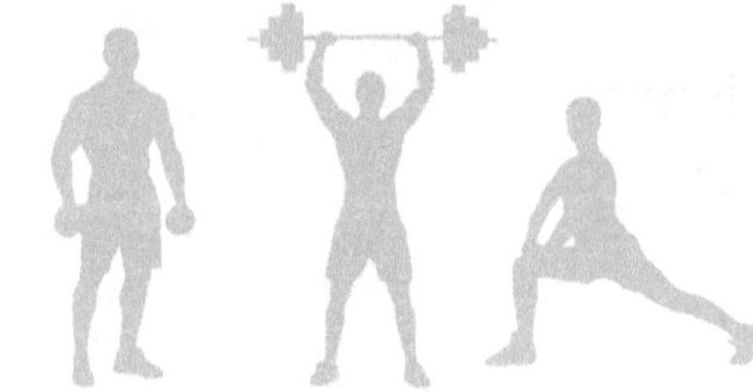

Name: ....

Date: ....

Time: ....

Warm-Up

ACTIVITY	TIME	REPS

 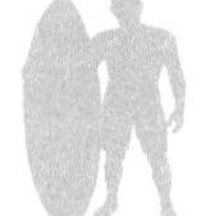 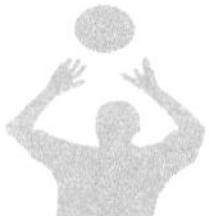 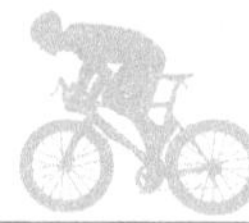

Cardio

ACTIVITY	DISTANCE	TIME	TARGET HEART RATE

Strength Training

EXERCISE	SET ONE WEIGHT/REPS	SET TWO WEIGHT/REPS	SET THREE WEIGHT/REPS

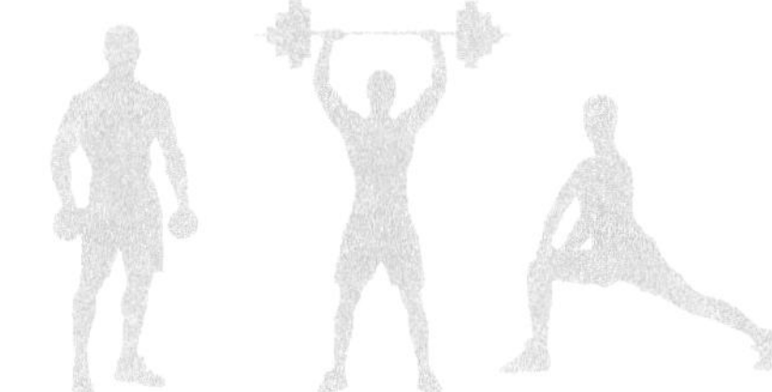

Warm-Up

ACTIVITY	TIME	REPS

 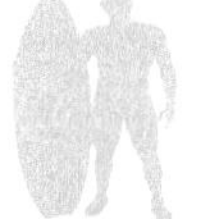 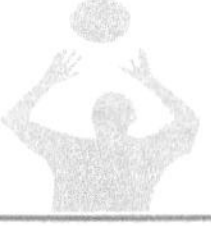 

Cardio

ACTIVITY	DISTANCE	TIME	TARGET HEART RATE

Strength Training

EXERCISE	SET ONE WEIGHT/REPS	SET TWO WEIGHT/REPS	SET THREE WEIGHT/REPS

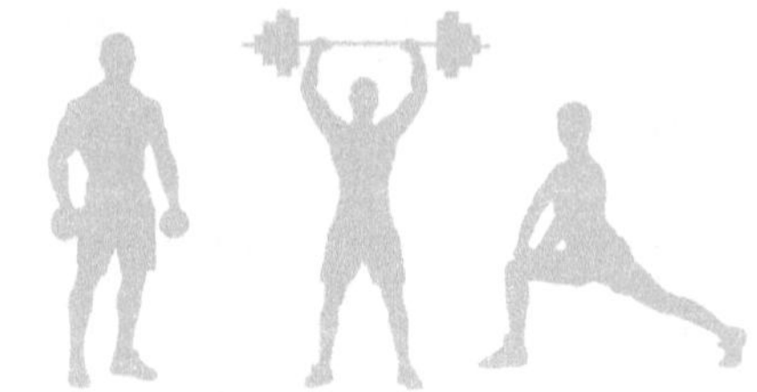

Name: ....

Date: ....

Time: ....

Warm-Up

ACTIVITY	TIME	REPS

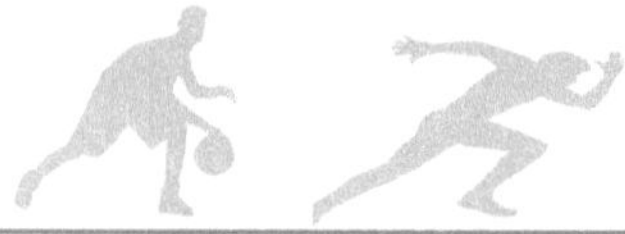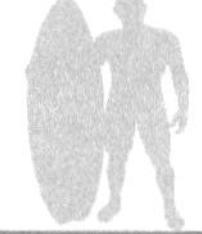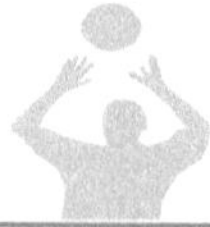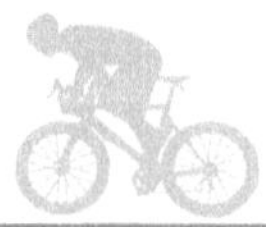

Cardio

ACTIVITY	DISTANCE	TIME	TARGET HEART RATE

Strength Training

EXERCISE	SET ONE WEIGHT/REPS	SET TWO WEIGHT/REPS	SET THREE WEIGHT/REPS

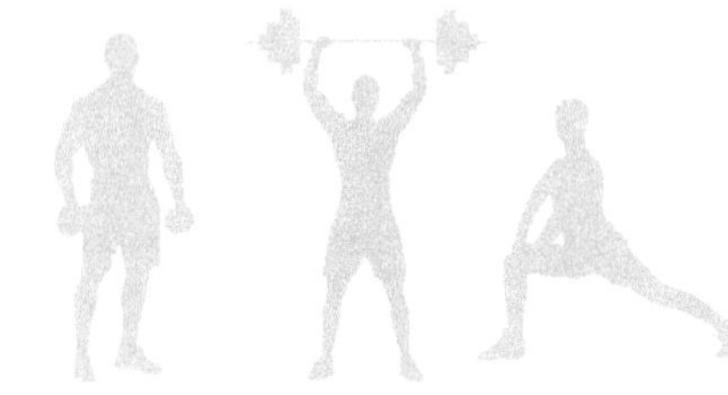

Name: ....

Date: ....

Time: ....

Warm-Up

ACTIVITY	TIME	REPS

Cardio

ACTIVITY	DISTANCE	TIME	TARGET HEART RATE

Strength Training

EXERCISE	SET ONE WEIGHT/REPS	SET TWO WEIGHT/REPS	SET THREE WEIGHT/REPS

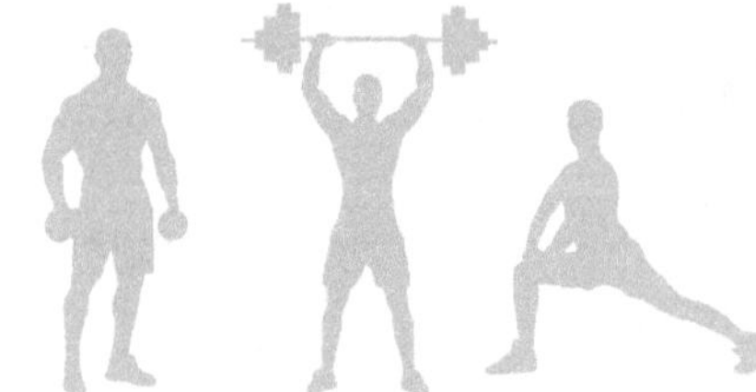

Name: ....

Date: ....

Time: ....

Warm-Up

ACTIVITY	TIME	REPS

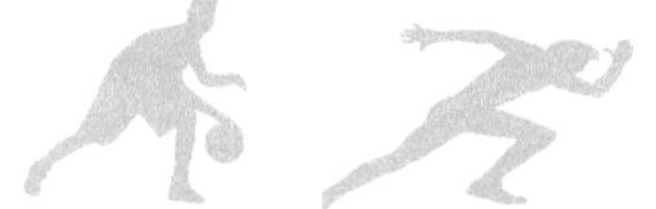 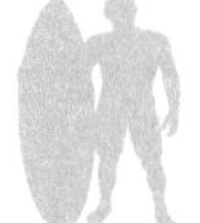 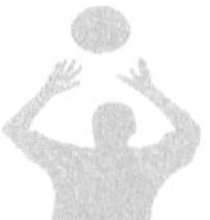 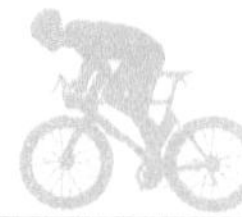

Cardio

ACTIVITY	DISTANCE	TIME	TARGET HEART RATE

Strength Training

EXERCISE	SET ONE WEIGHT/REPS	SET TWO WEIGHT/REPS	SET THREE WEIGHT/REPS

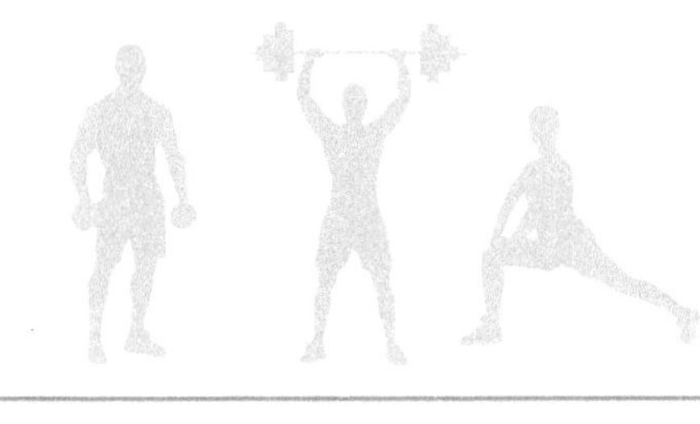

Name: ....

Date: ....

Time: ....

Warm-Up

ACTIVITY	TIME	REPS

Cardio

ACTIVITY	DISTANCE	TIME	TARGET HEART RATE

Strength Training

EXERCISE	SET ONE WEIGHT/REPS	SET TWO WEIGHT/REPS	SET THREE WEIGHT/REPS

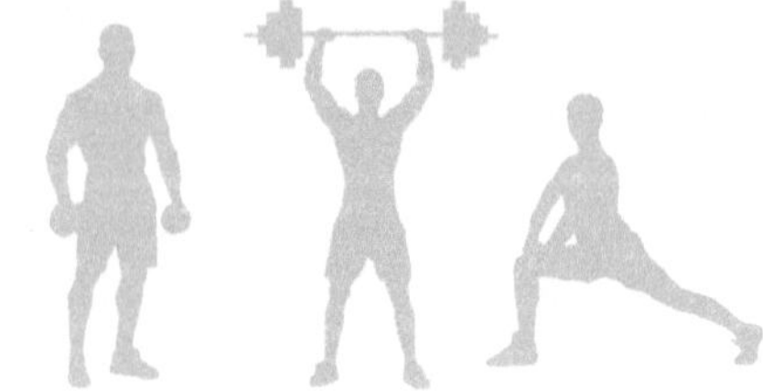

Name: ....

Date: ....

Time: ....

Warm-Up

ACTIVITY	TIME	REPS

 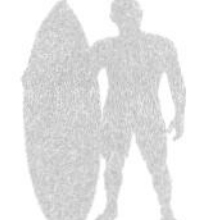 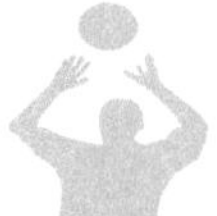 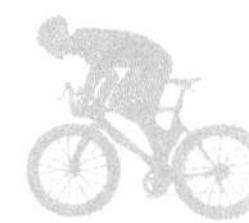

Cardio

ACTIVITY	DISTANCE	TIME	TARGET HEART RATE

Strength Training

EXERCISE	SET ONE WEIGHT/REPS	SET TWO WEIGHT/REPS	SET THREE WEIGHT/REPS

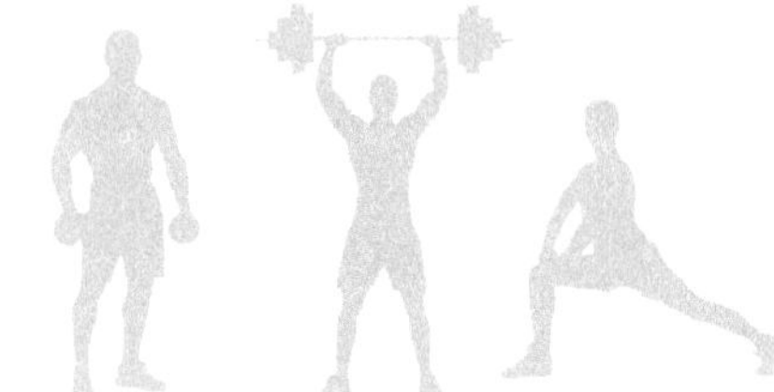

Name: ....

Date: ....

Time: ....

Warm-Up

ACTIVITY	TIME	REPS

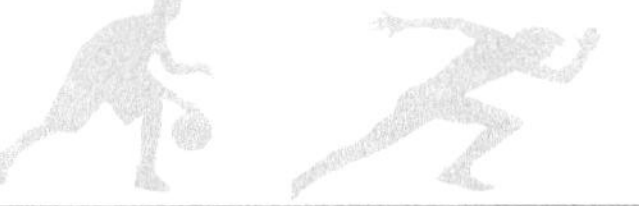 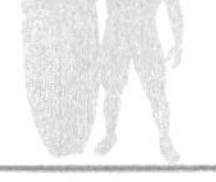 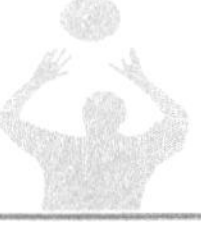 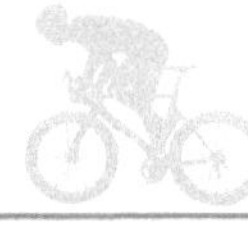

Cardio

ACTIVITY	DISTANCE	TIME	TARGET HEART RATE

Strength Training

EXERCISE	SET ONE WEIGHT/REPS	SET TWO WEIGHT/REPS	SET THREE WEIGHT/REPS

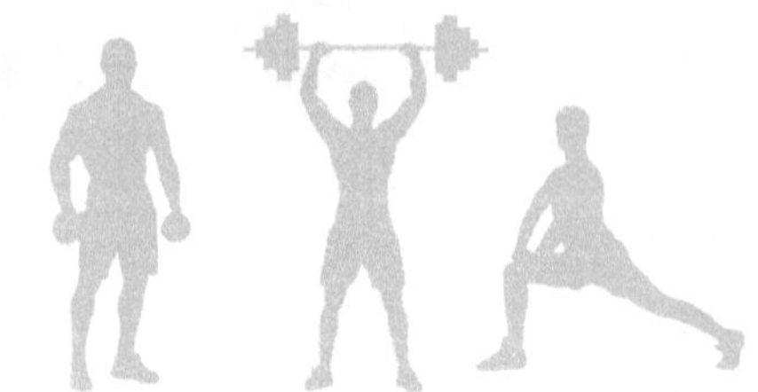

Name: ....

Date: ....

Time: ....

Warm-Up

ACTIVITY	TIME	REPS

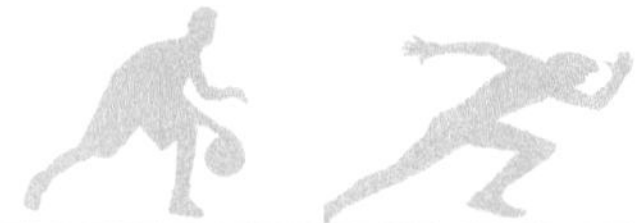 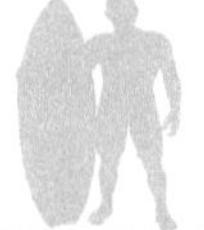 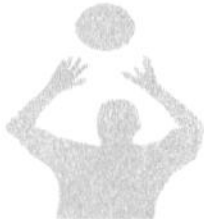 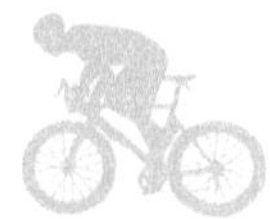

Cardio

ACTIVITY	DISTANCE	TIME	TARGET HEART RATE

Strength Training

EXERCISE	SET ONE WEIGHT/REPS	SET TWO WEIGHT/REPS	SET THREE WEIGHT/REPS

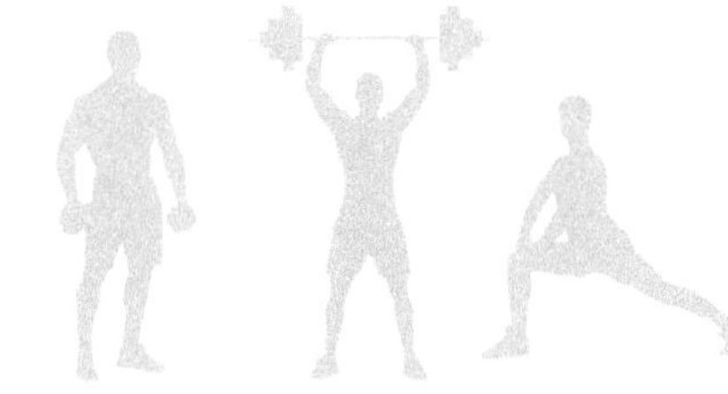

Name: ....

Date: ....

Time: ....

Warm-Up

ACTIVITY	TIME	REPS

Cardio

ACTIVITY	DISTANCE	TIME	TARGET HEART RATE

Strength Training

EXERCISE	SET ONE WEIGHT/REPS	SET TWO WEIGHT/REPS	SET THREE WEIGHT/REPS

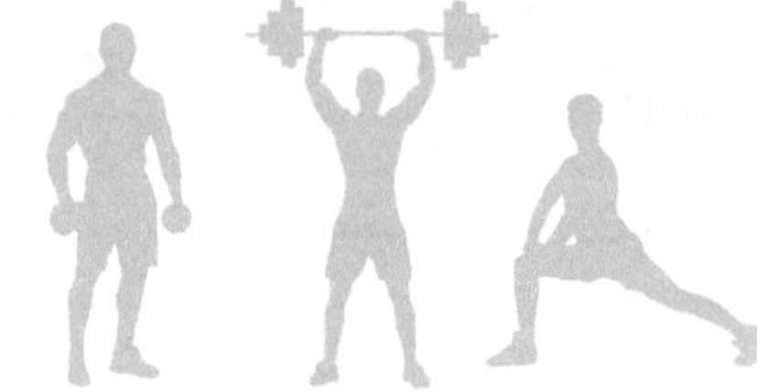

Name: ....

Date: ....

Time: ....

Warm-Up

ACTIVITY	TIME	REPS

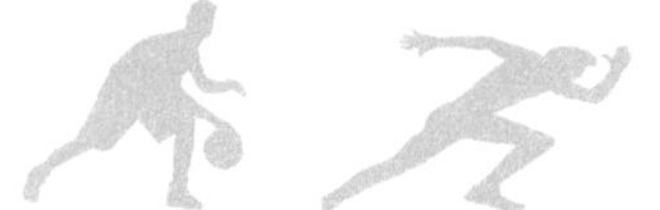 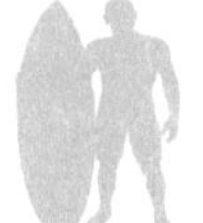 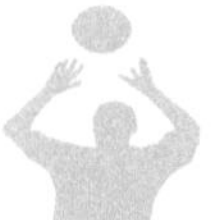 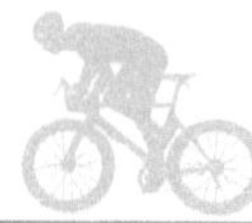

Cardio

ACTIVITY	DISTANCE	TIME	TARGET HEART RATE

Strength Training

EXERCISE	SET ONE WEIGHT/REPS	SET TWO WEIGHT/REPS	SET THREE WEIGHT/REPS

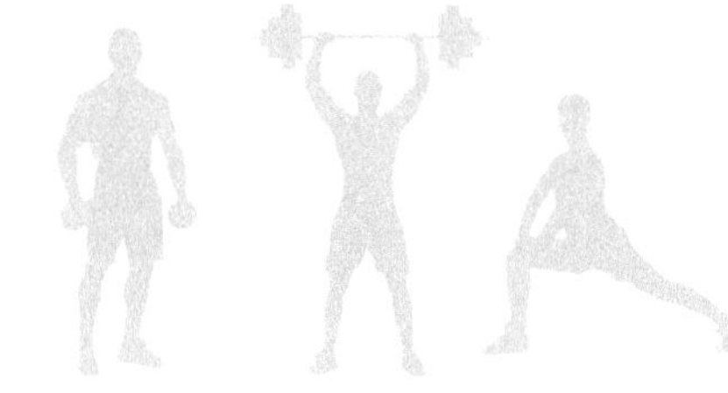

Name: ....

Date: ....

Time: ....

Warm-Up

ACTIVITY	TIME	REPS

Cardio

ACTIVITY	DISTANCE	TIME	TARGET HEART RATE

Strength Training

EXERCISE	SET ONE WEIGHT/REPS	SET TWO WEIGHT/REPS	SET THREE WEIGHT/REPS

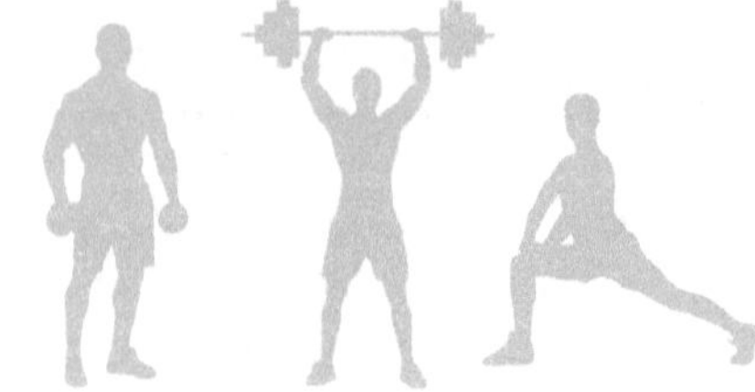

Name: ....

Date: ....

Time: ....

Warm-Up

ACTIVITY	TIME	REPS

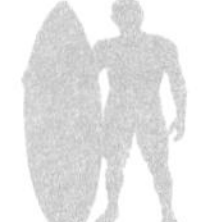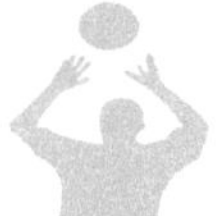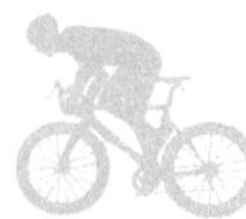

Cardio

ACTIVITY	DISTANCE	TIME	TARGET HEART RATE

Strength Training

EXERCISE	SET ONE WEIGHT/REPS	SET TWO WEIGHT/REPS	SET THREE WEIGHT/REPS

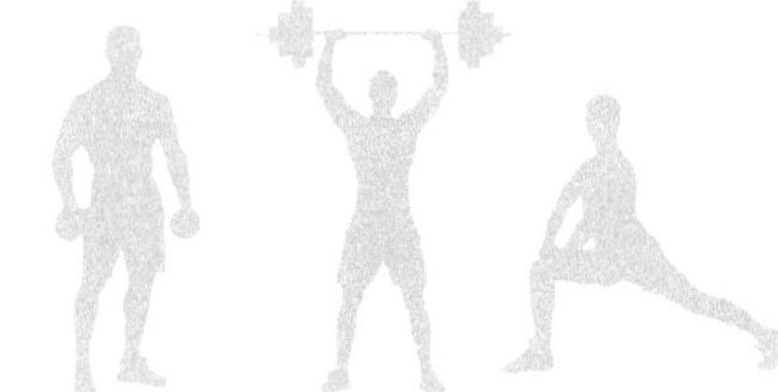

Name: ....

Date: ....

Time: ....

Warm-Up

ACTIVITY	TIME	REPS

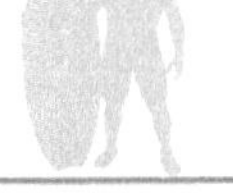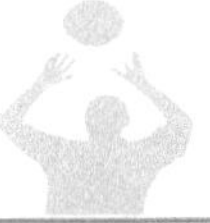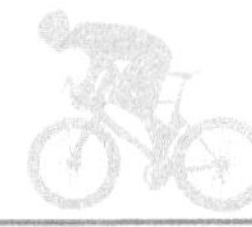

Cardio

ACTIVITY	DISTANCE	TIME	TARGET HEART RATE

Strength Training

EXERCISE	SET ONE WEIGHT/REPS	SET TWO WEIGHT/REPS	SET THREE WEIGHT/REPS

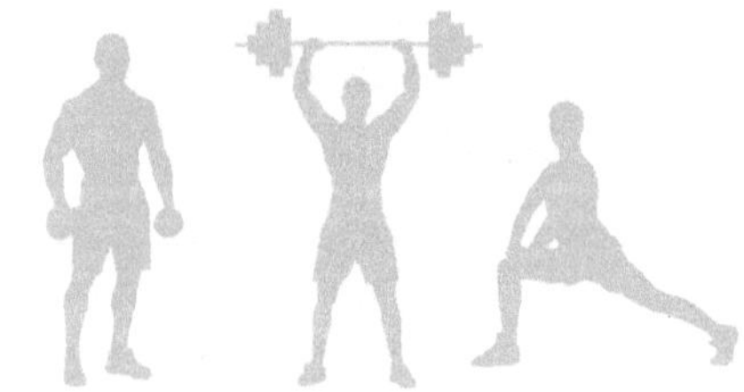

Name: ....

Date: ....

Time: ....

Warm-Up

ACTIVITY	TIME	REPS

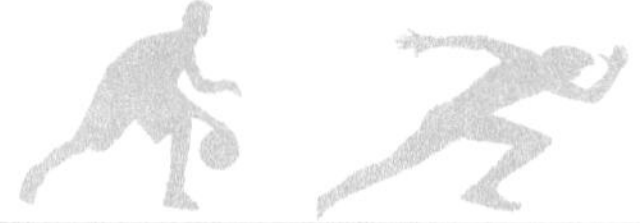 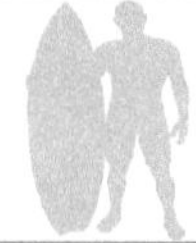 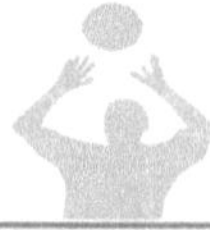 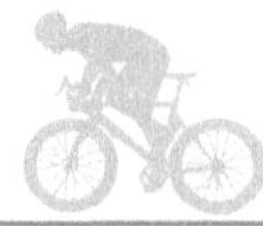

Cardio

ACTIVITY	DISTANCE	TIME	TARGET HEART RATE

Strength Training

EXERCISE	SET ONE WEIGHT/REPS	SET TWO WEIGHT/REPS	SET THREE WEIGHT/REPS

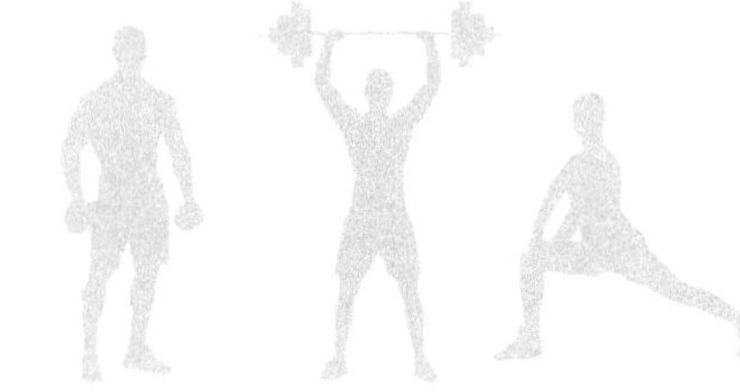

Name: ....

Date: ....

Time: ....

Warm-Up

ACTIVITY	TIME	REPS

Cardio

ACTIVITY	DISTANCE	TIME	TARGET HEART RATE

Strength Training

EXERCISE	SET ONE WEIGHT/REPS	SET TWO WEIGHT/REPS	SET THREE WEIGHT/REPS

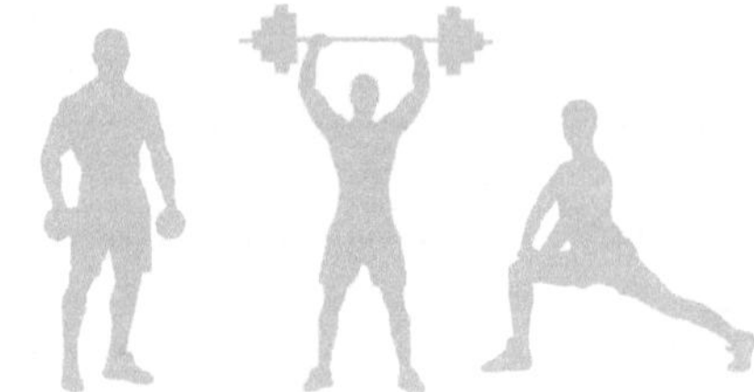

Name: ....

Date: ....

Time: ....

Warm-Up

ACTIVITY	TIME	REPS

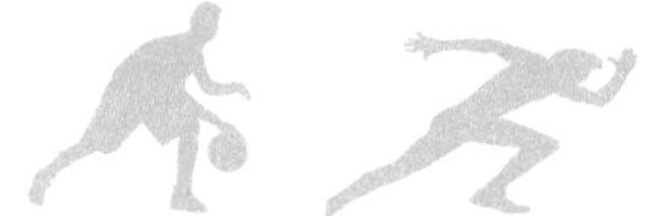 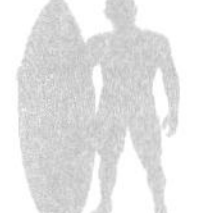 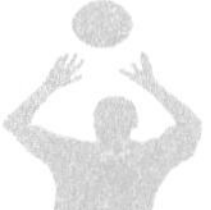 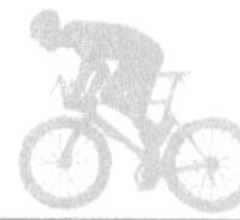

Cardio

ACTIVITY	DISTANCE	TIME	TARGET HEART RATE

Strength Training

EXERCISE	SET ONE WEIGHT/REPS	SET TWO WEIGHT/REPS	SET THREE WEIGHT/REPS

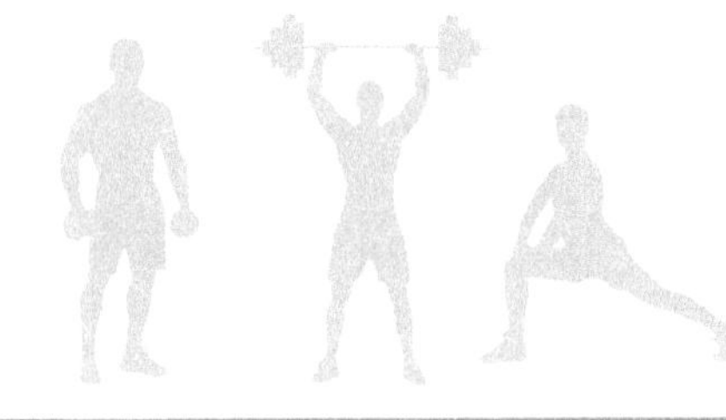

Warm-Up

ACTIVITY	TIME	REPS

Cardio

ACTIVITY	DISTANCE	TIME	TARGET HEART RATE

Strength Training

EXERCISE	SET ONE WEIGHT/REPS	SET TWO WEIGHT/REPS	SET THREE WEIGHT/REPS

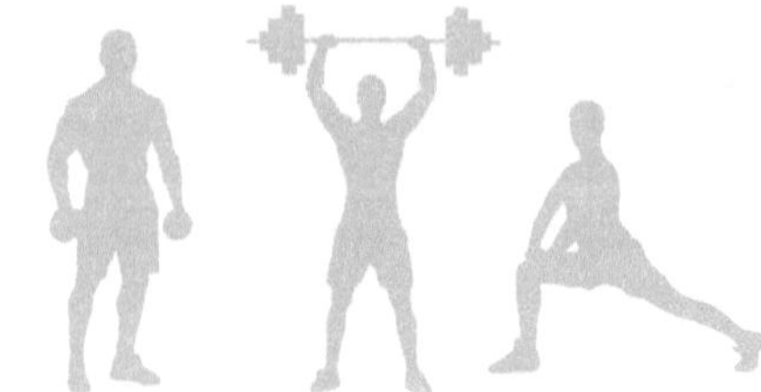

Name: ....

Date: ....

Time: ....

Warm-Up

ACTIVITY	TIME	REPS

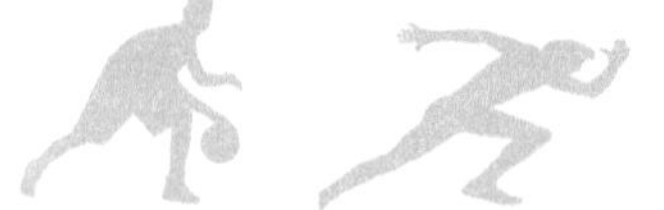 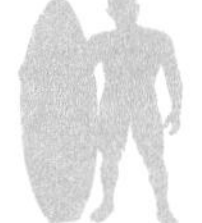 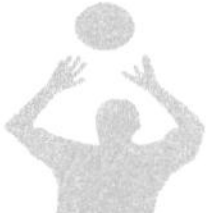 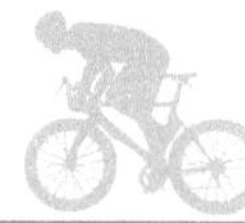

Cardio

ACTIVITY	DISTANCE	TIME	TARGET HEART RATE

Strength Training

EXERCISE	SET ONE WEIGHT/REPS	SET TWO WEIGHT/REPS	SET THREE WEIGHT/REPS

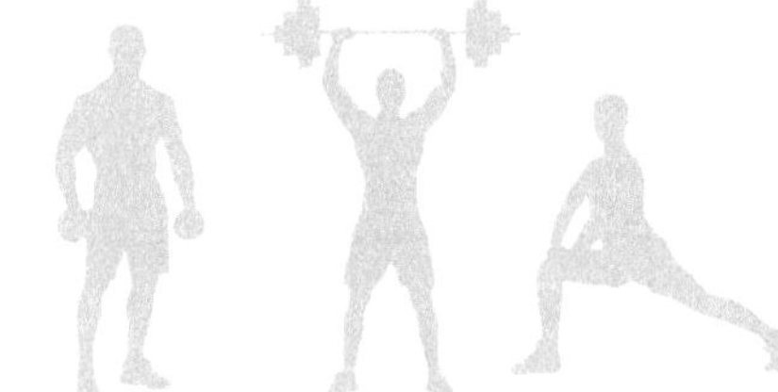

Name: ....

Date: ....

Time: ....

Warm-Up

ACTIVITY	TIME	REPS

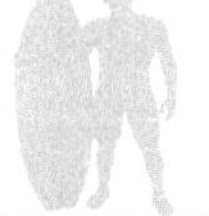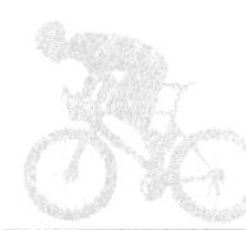

Cardio

ACTIVITY	DISTANCE	TIME	TARGET HEART RATE

Strength Training

EXERCISE	SET ONE WEIGHT/REPS	SET TWO WEIGHT/REPS	SET THREE WEIGHT/REPS

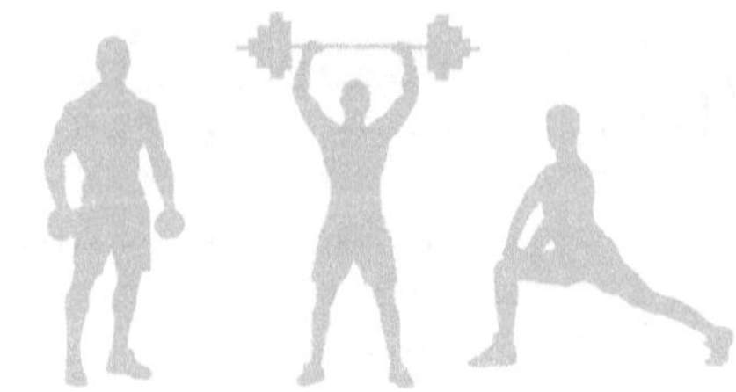

Warm-Up

ACTIVITY	TIME	REPS

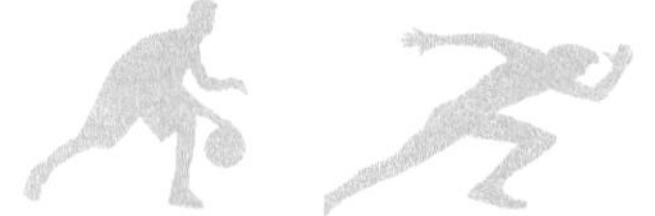  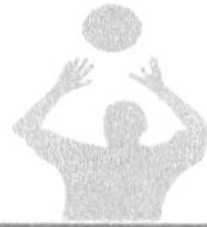 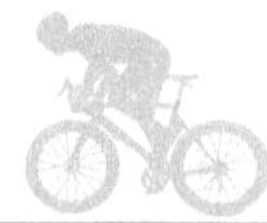

Cardio

ACTIVITY	DISTANCE	TIME	TARGET HEART RATE

Strength Training

EXERCISE	SET ONE WEIGHT/REPS	SET TWO WEIGHT/REPS	SET THREE WEIGHT/REPS

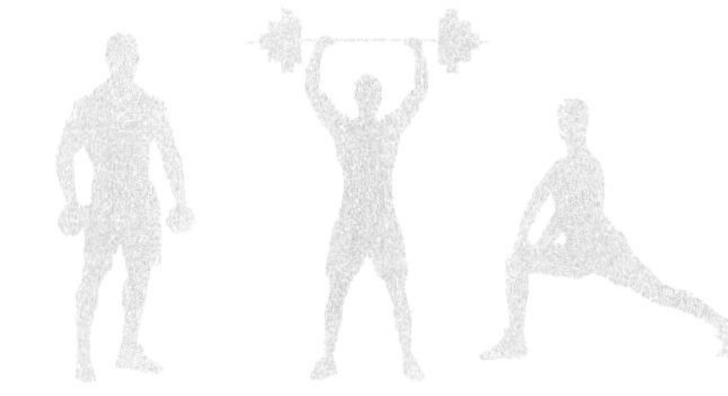

Name: ....

Date: ....

Time: ....

Warm-Up

ACTIVITY	TIME	REPS

Cardio

ACTIVITY	DISTANCE	TIME	TARGET HEART RATE

Strength Training

EXERCISE	SET ONE WEIGHT/REPS	SET TWO WEIGHT/REPS	SET THREE WEIGHT/REPS

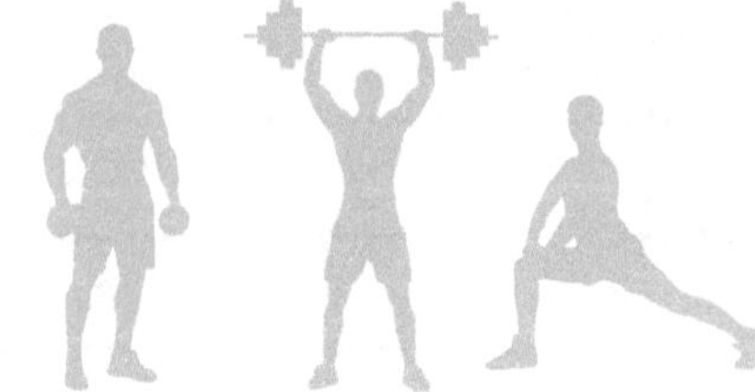

Name: ....

Date: ....

Time: ....

Warm-Up

ACTIVITY	TIME	REPS

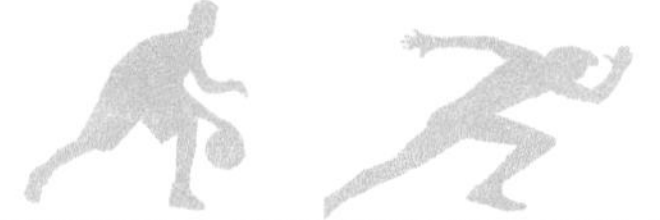 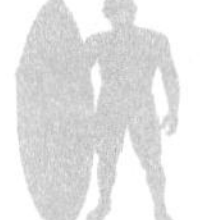 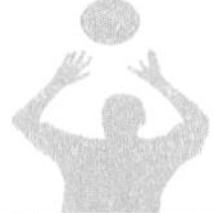 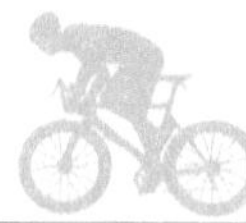

Cardio

ACTIVITY	DISTANCE	TIME	TARGET HEART RATE

Strength Training

EXERCISE	SET ONE WEIGHT/REPS	SET TWO WEIGHT/REPS	SET THREE WEIGHT/REPS

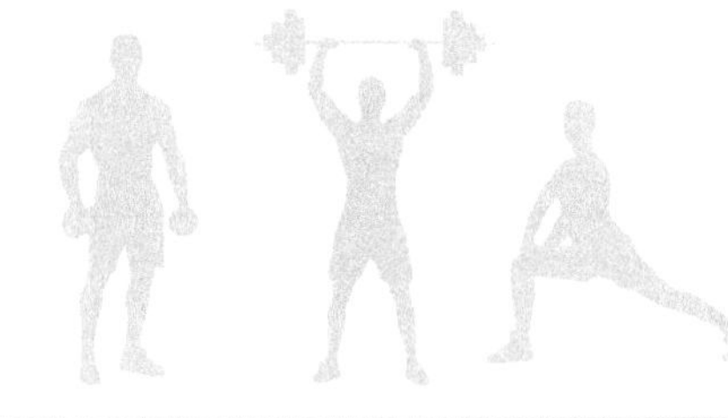

Name: ……………………………..

Date: ……………………………..

Time: ……………………………..

Warm-Up

ACTIVITY	TIME	REPS

Cardio

ACTIVITY	DISTANCE	TIME	TARGET HEART RATE

Strength Training

EXERCISE	SET ONE WEIGHT/REPS	SET TWO WEIGHT/REPS	SET THREE WEIGHT/REPS

Weekly Weight Tracker

Name...............................
Starting Weight................
Target Weight...................

DATE	CURRENT WEIGHT	WEIGHT LOST	WEIGHT GAINED

Weekly Weight Tracker

Name..............................
Starting Weight................
Target Weight...................

DATE	CURRENT WEIGHT	WEIGHT LOST	WEIGHT GAINED

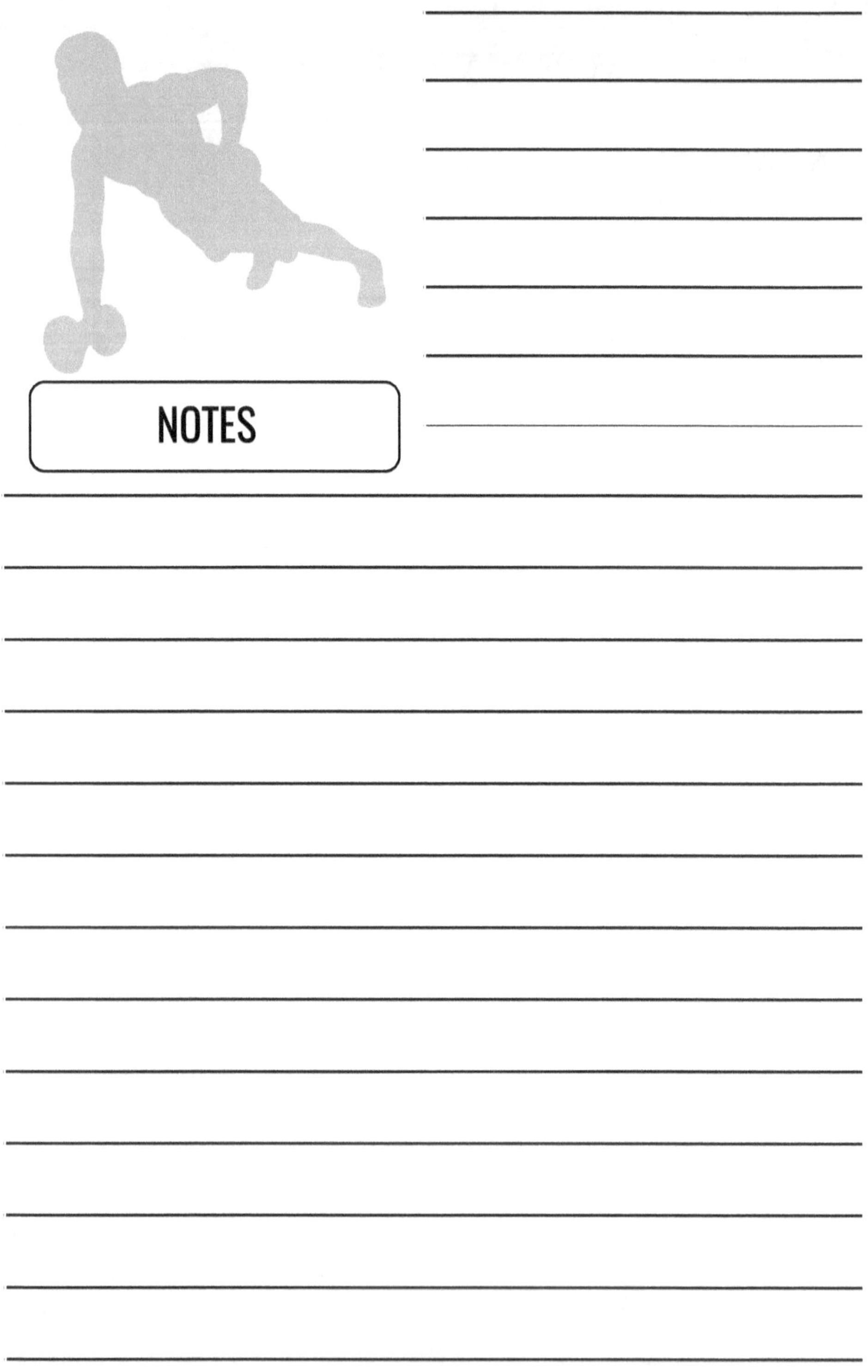

NOTES

NOTES

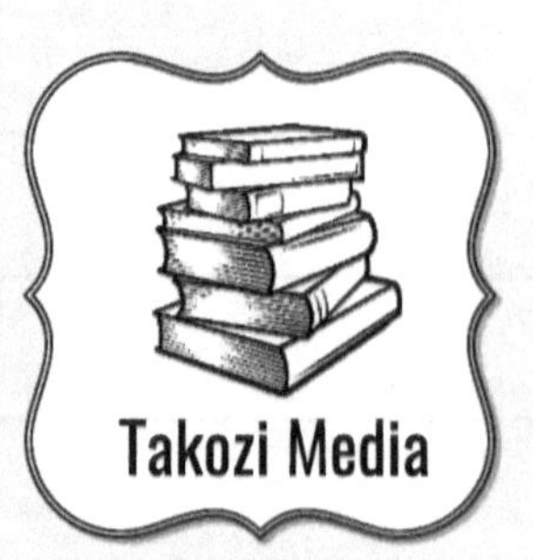
Takozi Media